THE CONTRACEPTION DECEPTION

Praise for *The Contraception Deception*

"Witty, provocative and informative, this vademecum for a new generation, proud to affirm allegiance to sound Catholic principles, will delight and challenge its readers. A book that is eminently readable, I am pleased to recommend it with enthusiasm."

—Archbishop Terrence Prendergast, S.J.
Archbishop of Ottawa

"There is a lot of great discussion about respect for women these days, but it's all stymied by the fact that our culture holds views about sexuality that are deeply degrading to females. *The Contraception Deception* takes an important step in helping us develop a view of sexual morality that leads to better relationships and true empowerment for women."

—Jennifer Fulwiler
SiriusXM radio host and author of *One Beautiful Dream*

"Patrick Coffin is an excellent educator who has the rare gift of being engaging without lapsing into the loose colloquialisms and self-conscious hipness that often mars well-intended articulations of the Church's sexual teachings. Faithful and solidly written, with ample historical background, *The Contraception Deception* provides a lucid and engaging defense of the Church's teachings against contraception that should be helpful to couples as well as those wishing to sharpen their skills in defending the faith."

—Dawn Eden Goldstein
Assistant Professor at Holy Apostles College and Seminary and award-winning author of *The Thrill of the Chaste*

"In *The Contraception Deception*, Patrick Coffin presents a clear and compelling case for the timeless teaching of the Church on contraception. Coffin demonstrates the beauty, power, and joy that is possible in marital sexual love when a couple does not separate what God has joined—their union expressing life-giving love."

—KIMBERLY HAHN
Bestselling author and speaker

"I love *The Contraception Deception* because it's that rare book on sexual matters that can be recommended to anyone—whether or not one is a member of the Catholic tribe. Polarizing misconceptions about life and love, babies and bonding, caring and carnality, dissolve in mutual understanding and respect. Coffin's words are candid but never crass. He embraces natural law while rejecting legalism and he doesn't avoid difficult situations or escape into relativism. This book is a great guide in a conversation that is almost always wildly misguided."

—AL KRESTA
President/CEO Ave Maria Communications
and host of *Kresta in the Afternoon*

"Sex is deeply important to everyone, everywhere, and yet, as our decadent popular culture amply demonstrates, most moderns don't really understand sex at all beyond the pleasure it gives. Its deeper purpose and meanings are left largely unexamined nowadays, which is why *The Contraception Deception* is so timely and important. Coffin unveils the 'why?' and 'for whom?' of sex clearly and convincingly, without polemics or moralizing."

—PATRICK MADRID
Host of *The Patrick Madrid Show* on Relevant Radio

"A fast-paced, easy to read, intelligent conversation about one of the most misunderstood Church teachings. Consider this a must for your personal library, whether you agree with *Humanae Vitae* or not."

—Pia de Solenni, SThD
Chancellor of the Diocese of Orange and
Theological Advisor to the Bishop

"*The Contraception Deception* is concise, clear, and charitable. No one brings these qualities to the most contentious issue of our time more effectively than Patrick Coffin. If you want to know the why behind the what of the Church's teaching on contraception, *this* is a must read."

—Chris Stefanick
Author, speaker, and founder of Real Life Catholic

"I firmly believe that Catholic teaching on contraception will one day be vindicated around the world. Patrick Coffin's own journey from dissent to discovery will resonate with a whole generation who were really never invited to 'come and see' this sublime vision of sexuality and Christian marriage."

—Christopher West
Author, speaker, and co-founder of
the Theology of the Body Institute

THE CONTRACEPTION DECEPTION

CATHOLIC TEACHING ON BIRTH CONTROL

Second Edition

Patrick Coffin

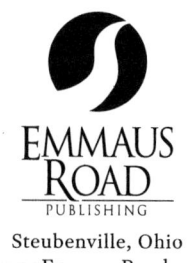

EMMAUS ROAD
PUBLISHING

Steubenville, Ohio
www.EmmausRoad.org

Emmaus Road Publishing
1468 Parkview Circle
Steubenville, Ohio 43952

©2010, 2018 Patrick Coffin
All rights reserved. First edition 2010, printed under title *Sex au Naturel*
Second edition 2018, printed with new title *The Contraception Deception*
Printed in the United States of America

Library of Congress Control no: 2018938170
ISBN: 978-1-947792-80-7

Unless otherwise noted, Scripture quotations are taken from The Revised Standard Version Second Catholic Edition (Ignatius Edition) Copyright © 2006 by the Division of Christian Education of the National Council of the Churches of Christ in the United States of America. Used by permission. All rights reserved.

Excerpts from the *Catechism of the Catholic Church*, second edition, copyright © 2000, Libreria Editrice Vaticana--United States Conference of Catholic Bishops, Washington, D.C.

Cover image: *The Kiss* (1907–1908), Gustav Klimt,
The Belvedere Museum, Vienna, Austria

Cover design and layout by Margaret Ryland

+

To the memory of Naomi Rose Coffin
(September 14, 2006—September 29, 2006)

For we are also what we have lost, amorcito.

Contents

Foreword	xiii
Acknowledgements	xvii
Abbreviations	xxi
Introduction	1
1. How We Got Here	15
2. Escape from Dissent	29
3. Who's Your Daddy?	43
4. Birth Control in the Bible	53
5. Birth Control and the Blessed Trinity	81
6. Contraception and the Natural Law	95
7. Answers to the Pop Quiz	113
8. The Population Bomb Myth	125
9. Planned Barrenhood	139
10. Made, Not Begotten	155
11. N.F.P. vs. A.B.C.	171
Epilogue	183
Appendix	191

FOREWORD

I am very happy to have read this book because otherwise I would have to write it myself. (I write the books I wish someone else would write, but they don't, so I do.)

This is *exactly* the book that needs to be written today, for:

(1) It's about the lynchpin and foundation of the Sexual Revolution, which is the most radical and life-changing revolution since Christianity. Without contraception, no Sexual Revolution. The Pill has changed more lives more radically than the printing press, the steam engine, the assembly line, or the atomic bomb.

(2) It's about the most controversial and controverted Church teaching in history. No official document has ever generated more "dissent" than *Humanae Vitae*.

(3) It's written for everyone, not just for scholars.

(4) But it's not "popular" in the usual sense of dumbed down or shallow.

(5) And it's *complete*. Coffin covers the waterfront. Nothing is missing. (Just look at the Table of Contents.) The author has read and digested all the vast

literature on the subject and has served it to us in a meal of well-ordered, edible courses.

George Weigel famously and rightly called John Paul the Great's "Theology of the Body" a "theological time bomb." It is the Church's answer to the Sexual Revolution. It's profound, and it's beautiful, and it's human, and it's winsome. It's the Big Picture behind *Humanae Vitae*.

The Church has always come up with what the time most desperately needs. Creeds come in response to heresies. We can even thank God for heresies ("*O felix culpa!*") because without them, we would not have the Creeds. The Church has always practiced St. Paul's principle "Test everything; hold fast what is good." (1 Thess 5:21, RSV)

But John Paul's writings on the Theology of the Body are dense, and long. Christopher West has "translated" them into much more accessible prose. But even his magisterial work is still fairly long and not an "easy read" (though it is deeply rewarding and potentially life-changing). Patrick Coffin has done for Christopher West what Christopher West has done for John Paul II.

Do you think there is nothing but blind obedience and "dead orthodoxy" behind support of *Humanae Vitae*? You won't think that after you read this book.

Do you want to believe what the Church teaches but find it hard? You won't find it hard after you read this book.

Do you believe it but merely out of loyalty, without understanding it, either instinctively, or rationally, or sympathetically? You won't believe in that way after you read this book.

Do you believe *Humanae Vitae* but despair of explaining it to the average "dissenter"? You won't despair after you read this book. (And you'll have plenty of opportunities to explain it. For "the average dissenter" means the vast majority of Europeans and North Americans today, Catholics as well as non-Catholics.)

Are you confused and open-minded about the whole issue? You won't be after you read this book.

Are you bored with the whole issue? (Why have you read this far, then?) You won't be after you read this book.

Do you think the issue is peripheral, accidental, secondary, dispensable? You won't think that after you read this book.

Do you think the Church's instinctive attitude toward sex is a frown? Do you think *The Catholic Sex Book* would be a blank book? You won't think that after you read this book.

So read this book.

—*Peter Kreeft*

ACKNOWLEDGEMENTS

This book began life as notes for a public lecture given at Pierce College in Los Angeles, sponsored by LA Jewish Family Services and the Encore-Oasis Adult Education Program. It was then fed and reared by many people, by their helpful criticism of the manuscript, by giving research leads, or by making their formidable brains available for picking: the late Dr. Germain Grisez; the late Msgr. Vincent Foy (the longest serving priest in Canadian history); Jimmy Akin; Fr. Lambert Greenan, OP; Dr. Gregory Polito, MD, KM; Dr. Patrick Lee; Domenico Bettinelli; Dr. Terry Vanderheyden, ND; Albert Faraj; Fr. James Mallon; Judy Savoy; and the indulgent staff at the Joanne D'Arcy Canyon Country Library.

The teaching of the Catholic Church against contraception is winning friends and influencing more people today than its early enemies in the 1960s could have predicted, thanks to a wave of orthodox defenders and teachers of the Catholic sexual ethic. The primal force within the Church behind that wave was the late Pope St. John Paul the Great through his encyclicals, exhortations, public speeches, and, particularly, one-hundred-and-twenty-nine weekly General

Audiences he gave from 1979 to 1984, which became known as the Theology of the Body.

I have been inspired by the skilled surfers of that wave and by those who early on defended this perennial teaching of Christ. These include Dr. Janet E. Smith, who loved *Humanae Vitae* before loving *Humanae Vitae* was cool and who has done more than anyone in the English-speaking world to make it better loved; Christopher West, the exuberant ambassador of John Paul II's Theology of the Body; Canadian philosopher and pro-life lion Dr. Donald DeMarco; the late Fr. John McGoey, SFM, of Toronto, whose writings about emotional and sexual maturity should be required reading for all serious Catholics; the dynamic duo of Scott and Kimberly Hahn, for their contributions to a new familial explication of covenant theology; John and Sheila Kippley, pioneering founders of the Couple to Couple League and promoters of the Sympto-Thermal Method of natural family planning; Dr. Thomas Hilgers, MD, discoverer and developer of NaProTechnology and the Creighton Model FertilityCareTM System; and Drs. John and Evelyn Billings, original co-developers of the Ovulation Method, the first truly modern natural family planning technology.

To change the surfing metaphor, the above individuals hacked through layers of thick underbrush with their respective machetes to reveal a serene and beautiful clearing known as the Catholic sexual ethic. My small contribution to their hard work—work that was often derided when it wasn't being ignored—is to show up and point out the gorgeous scenery.

The late Sr. Therese Moore, SC, professor of English at Mount Saint Vincent University in Halifax, Nova Scotia, was the first to turn my love for words into a love for stringing them together. The weaknesses in the following strings belong to me alone.

ACKNOWLEDGMENTS

A special word of gratitude goes to Chris Erickson of Emmaus Road Publishing, who shepherded the revised iteration of the book, and to editor Melissa Girard, whose incisive comments and insights made for improvements all around. Kudos to the rest of the support staff at Emmaus Road, and to its founder, my good friend Dr. Scott Hahn. If publishers were medals, your lot would be gold. Lest I forget, thanks as well to Mary Melton for her holy persistence in getting me to introduce *Humanae Vitae* to a non-Christian audience in the first place.

Finally, without the support of my wife Mariella, the witness of fifty-eight years of marriage of my parents, Jack and Marian Coffin, and the unutterable patience of my daughters, Mariclare and Sophia, what follows would have just stayed a good idea.

ABBREVIATIONS

Old Testament

Gen	Genesis	Song	Song of Solomon
Exod	Exodus	Wis	Wisdom
Lev	Leviticus	Sir	Sirach
Num	Numbers	Isa	Isaiah
Deut	Deuteronomy	Jer	Jeremiah
Josh	Joshua	Lam	Lamentations
Judg	Judges	Bar	Baruch
Ruth	Ruth	Ezek	Ezekiel
1 Sam	1 Samuel	Dan	Daniel
2 Sam	2 Samuel	Hos	Hosea
1 Kgs	1 Kings	Joel	Joel
2 Kgs	2 Kings	Amos	Amos
1 Chr	1 Chronicles	Obad	Obadiah
2 Chr	2 Chronicles	Jonah	Jonah
Ezra	Ezra	Mic	Micah
Neh	Nehemiah	Nah	Nahum
Tob	Tobit	Hab	Habakkuk
Jdt	Judith	Zeph	Zephaniah
Esth	Esther	Hag	Haggai
Job	Job	Zech	Zechariah
Ps	Psalms	Mal	Malachi
Prov	Proverbs	1 Macc	1 Maccabees
Eccl	Ecclesiastes	2 Macc	2 Maccabees

New Testament		Church Documents	
Matt	Matthew	CC	*Casti Connubii*
Mark	Mark	DV	*Dei Verbum*
Luke	Luke	FC	*Familiaris Consortio*
John	John	GS	*Gaudium et Spes*
Acts	Acts of the Apostles	HV	*Humanae Vitae*
Rom	Romans	CCC	Catechism of the Catholic Church
1 Cor	1 Corinthians		
2 Cor	2 Corinthians		
Gal	Galatians		
Eph	Ephesians		
Phil	Philippians		
Col	Colossians		
1 Thess	1 Thessalonians		
2 Thess	2 Thessalonians		
1 Tim	1 Timothy		
2 Tim	2 Timothy		
Tit	Titus		
Phil	Philemon		
Heb	Hebrews		
Jas	James		
1 Pet	1 Peter		
2 Pet	2 Peter		
1 John	1 John		
2 John	2 John		
3 John	3 John		
Jude	Jude		
Rev	Revelation		

Introduction

"SEX AU NATUREL" IN THE CROSSHAIRS

Sometimes the march of time turns into a sprint. In the eight years since the first edition of this book came out under the title *Sex Au Naturel: What It Is and Why It's Good For Your Marriage,* that sprint has at times felt more like a mad dash. Toward what destination? Whether off a cliff into chaos or into the warmth of a sunny utopia depends upon your attitude toward what human sexuality means or is supposed to mean.

And this explains the rationale for the new edition of this book, which originally hit Amazon on March 25, 2010—providentially, the Solemnity of the Annunciation. While I frankly didn't expect so many five-star reviews, it seems my treatment of the Catholic Church's teaching on contraception had hit a nerve, and I began to be asked to speak about it at conferences and in secular media outlets. Most people simply had never come across a defense of something deemed so *déclassé*, if not outright offensive to "pious" secular ears.

In 1929, a year before the Anglican communion overturned two-thousand years of Christian opposition to contraception, the English writer G. K. Chesterton wrote an under-appreciated book titled *The Thing: Why I Am a Catholic*, in which he takes aim at the linguistic subterfuges used by "birth controllers," like his contemporary Margaret Sanger.[1] "We can always convict such people of sentimentalism by their weakness for euphemism," he wrote. "The phrase they use is always softened and suited for journalistic appeals. They talk of free love when they mean something quite different, better defined as free lust. But being sentimentalists they feel bound to simper and coo over the word 'love.' They insist on talking about Birth Control when they mean less birth and no control."

Since the first edition, there have been some developments in the area of assistive reproductive technologies that I wanted to revisit. The time had also come to hone and somewhat reframe the overall line of argumentation. The Patient Protection and Affordable Care Act—quickly dubbed ObamaCare—was signed into law on March 23, 2010, just before the first edition of *Sex Au Naturel* went to print. Within a year, ObamaCare brought with it the Health and Human Services Mandate, which became known as the contraceptive mandate. All of a sudden, with the news of various lawsuits launched against the Obama Administration to defend freedom of conscience for employers, everyone was suddenly talking about contraception, but no one was talking about why the Church is against it.

With these legal affronts to religious freedom, the most controversial doctrine of the Catholic Church suddenly found itself in the crosshairs of a national debate, and the whole affair gave new life to the language of culture wars not

---

[1] Sanger is credited with coining the phrase birth control, which she embedded into the name of The American Birth Control League, which she founded in 1921, the forerunner to Planned Parenthood.

seen since then presidential candidate Patrick Buchanan first used it in his 1992 Republican Convention speech.

But the culture war is not primarily a war about the role of government or gun ownership or free speech. It is a war about sex, over what its meaning and purpose might be—or whether sex has any inherent meaning at all.

Before and after I launched my own podcast in 2017—*The Patrick Coffin Show,* along with a membership site devoted to faith and culture[2]—the inner logic of the sexual revolution as the main driver of the battle over American (hence, Western) culture became clearer. The clues were hiding in plain sight.

It is asked, often with irritation, "Why can't sex just be a brute fact, a neutral exchange of pleasure with only subjective meanings attached?" This is the prevailing view that has enabled the hook-up culture we see on college campuses and has led to social problems that are noticed by those who are, at this writing, outside the Faith. Dr. Jordan Peterson, professor of psychology and clinical psychologist (whom I have interviewed four times on *The Patrick Coffin Show*), is one of them. Dr. Peterson has unique insights into the ways in which contraception has disrupted the psycho-social relationship between the sexes and paved the way for the pornification of the culture.[3] As this book argues, the moral miasma surrounding contraception has nothing to do with religious dogma and everything to do with violating the very nature of healthy sexuality and its ends. Which is why there's a chapter on the natural law (Chapter Six).

If sex means whatever *I* say it means, then what limits can realistically be placed on its use? Anything goes, short

---

[2] The URL is www.patrickcoffin.media.
[3] The place to start is his website, www.jordanbpeterson.com.

of the infliction of pain? Too late. We're way past that. The sudden appearance of the highest-selling book in Amazon history testifies to a very broad societal acceptance of pain and humiliation as means toward adult entertainment (sic). That would be *Fifty Shades of Grey*. (As of this writing, its sequel *Fifty Shades Darker* ranks number five.)

The "Anything Goes, Except X, Which Is Obviously Beyond the Pale" principle has shown itself impossible to contain or implement in the real world. Examples are increasing and multiplying everywhere. Exact numbers are hard to come by, but Dr. Elizabeth Sheff, writing in *Psychology Today*, wrote that researcher Kelly Cookson's estimate of the number of couples who are, by mutual agreement, sexually non-monogamous is at 1.2 to 2.4 million.[4] Let's say that's grossly inflated (I happen to think it is). If it's off by 50 percent, that leaves over half a million. How many are actively working toward being legally recognized as married is unknown. *CBS News* reports that the State of Utah's strict monogamy laws have been challenged in recent years from some among the estimated 30,000 polygamists in Utah.[5] MercatorNet reports that three men in Thailand in 2015 and three women in Massachusetts in 2014 claimed to have "gotten married."[6]

Whether you think these last two cases are just publicity stunts is to miss the point. If marriage itself is redefined quite away from its three-thousand-year, transcultural prec-

---

[4] Elizabeth A. Sheff, PhD, "How Many Polyamorists Are There In the U.S.?" in *Psychology Today*, May 9, 2014. URL: https://www.psychologytoday.com/blog/the-polyamorists-next-door/201405/how-many-polyamorists-are-there-in-the-us.

[5] Associated Press report in CBSNews.com, March 29, 2017. URL: https://www.cbsnews.com/news/utah-gov-signs-law-aimed-at-polygamy/.

[6] Carolyn Moynihan, *MercatorNet*, March 9, 2015. URL: https://www.mercatornet.com/conjugality/view/the_advance_of_the_throuple/15750.

edent, on what logical basis do you limit it to two spouses?

Bestiality, you ask? Surely that is out of bounds. Again, sorry. (I hate to go here, but go we must.) In 2016, the Supreme Court of Canada ruled (six to one!) that sexual acts with animals are perfectly legal as long as there is no penetration, affirming the prior parliamentary vote of Prime Minister Justin Trudeau. The sexual abuse case that prompted the decision involves a stepfather violating his stepdaughter with a dog.[7] The only ones speaking up during the debate over this trial were animal rights activists. It didn't seem to occur to anyone to object on the basis of any injury to *human* dignity.

What is at stake in the debate over contraceptives is not merely which means of birth regulation are good and which are evil but the very question of who or what man is. If love and life—erotic intimacy and the coming to be of new human persons—can be intentionally disconnected, the logic is iron-clad and the consequences far exceed debates over family size and intramural squabbles over the fine points of moral theology among scholars. As we will see, figures as diverse as Mahatma Gandhi and Sigmund Freud saw that all sexual perversion is at its root contraceptive by definition.

Once the contraceptive mentality seeped into societal consciousness after World War II (with its mass refugee disruptions and the new research into developing a pill-based contraceptive), it was only a matter of time before all sorts of unforeseen outcomes began to emerge. But the real momentum toward the social and sexual chaos that announces itself in news headlines—the spread of no fault divorce, to the mainstreaming of pornography, down to the Hollywood #metoo campaign—first began with the large-scale dissent

---

[7] Full trial documents are available at https://scc-csc.lexum.com/scc-csc/scc-csc/en/item/15991/index.do.

inside Catholicism against the 1968 encyclical *Humanae Vitae* by Blessed Pope Paul VI.

This dissent from the norms of the most maligned, little-read encyclical in history led slowly but inexorably to the foundation-shaking redefinition of marriage itself, first in the Netherlands in 2001 and in America with the 2015 *Obergefell v. Hodges* Supreme Court decision. Other countries are rapidly following suit.

Obergefell is one more inevitable apotheosis of dissent from *Humanae Vitae*. Once sex had been redefined as an individualistic, even narcissistic (or whatever) affair between consenting adults, the drive toward acceptance of homosexual behavior began. It was a matter of time before the definition of marriage itself would be placed on the chopping block. And in lurching from march to mad dash, time has also brought us a whole new bundle of sexual confusions with the rise of the phenomenon of transgenderism. Again, if sex as an act is merely a bendy, pliable construct, then sex as a gender was next in line.

Set against the canvas of creation, and hence of pro-creation, the teaching of *Humanae Vitae* is easier to understand but still hard to explain. The challenge is compounded by the fact that two generations of Catholics (along with everyone else) have been conditioned to see birth control as an instrument of women's liberation, a panacea for marital strife, a fuel injection for sexual ecstasy, and a triumph of human ingenuity over cruel "Nature, red in tooth and claw."

Birth control bad for people? You might as well stroll the beaches in August with a bullhorn telling people to put away their sunscreen. Today birth control is no longer argued for; it is widely assumed to be a blessing. Condoms are a staple of late-night TV monologue jokes, are sold next to *Cosmopolitan* in the grocery express lane, and are part of the typical orientation tote bags given to college freshmen. The Pill (the only pill that gets a "the" in front of it) is dispensed by the tens of millions to ever younger and younger women, often without their parents' consent. Large families are seen by most people under forty as either the choice by ignorant Ozark inbreds, a self-administered curse, or possibly the attitude you'd find among Mormons. To say the least, large families are no longer viewed as signs of God's blessing.

This whole attitude has been the cultural default opinion for some time. Contrast this opinion with a snapshot of the previous default opinion, at least among Catholics. It's from a remarkable, if little-known, speech given in 1958 by Ven. Pope Pius XII to an organization called the Association for Large Families of Rome and Italy:

> The joy that comes from the plentiful blessings of God breaks out in a thousand different ways and there is no fear that it will end. The brows of these fathers and mothers may be burdened with cares, but there is never a trace of that inner shadow that betrays anxiety of conscience or fear of an irreparable return to loneliness; their youth never seems to fade away, as long as the sweet fragrance of a crib remains in the home, as long as the walls of the house echo to the silvery voices of children and grandchildren.[8]

Pop Quiz

The average person has no clear idea why the Catholic Church is opposed to contraception. Do you? Archbishop

---

[8] Pius XII, "Allocution to the Association for Large Families in Rome and Italy, January 19, 1958," *The Pope Speaks* 4 (Spring 1958): 363–64.

Fulton Sheen famously said that millions hate what they wrongly believe to be the Catholic Church. Millions also wrongly hate what they believe to be her teaching on contraception. If you disagree, try out this true-or-false quiz:

1) Protestants have always accepted contraception.
2) Mahatma Gandhi approved of contraception.
3) Sigmund Freud approved of contraception.
4) Contraceptives have always been legal in the United States.
5) More contraception leads to fewer abortions.
6) One can be a faithful Catholic and still contracept in good conscience.
7) The Pill is now medically safe for women.
8) The Rhythm Method is now called Natural Family Planning.
9) The Church teaches that women should have as many babies as possible.
10) The Catholic Church is opposed to all forms of birth regulation.
11) The Bible is silent on the matter of contraception.
12) Catholic teaching against contraception is fixed and cannot change.

(*Answers found in Chapter Seven*)

What Is at Stake

If you agree with the teaching of *Humanae Vitae*, that "each and every marital act must be open to new life" (no. 11), then, in the grand tradition of preaching to the choir, this revised edition will hopefully provide ammunition for those "friendly discussions" with family members or friends who think the teaching is nonsense (or worse). If you're not sure where you stand, what follows will hopefully help you see this teaching with a new set of eyes.

In this delicate arena, intellectual arguments alone are generally useless in the persuasion department. The subject matter relates as much to the will and to the heart as to the intellect.

For Catholic teaching against birth control asks that one be willing, when the occasion warrants, to keep in check one of the most imperious, at times unruly, appetites within the human person—the sexual urge. Our culture routinely identifies sex with love. Watch any Hollywood romantic comedy made since 1970 and you will find that fornication has been rebranded as a celluloid sacrament, love's highest expression.

Given the inherent pleasure in sex (which is God's idea) we are prone to fooling ourselves about what is and is not "love's highest expression." As Frank Sheed humorously quipped, "In no area is autokiddery so active than in the sexual."[9] To keep some of our appetites in proper order, we need extra help from the good Lord.

Therefore, this book has an evangelistic purpose. Given the bent of human nature toward its own cravings, its dread of admitting wrongdoing, and in consideration of our increasingly pornified culture, I believe the message of *Humanae Vitae* barely stands a chance of being understood, let alone embraced, without a singular grace from God. Without the help of that grace, the deck is rather stacked against seekers of truth. Yet the Truth Himself is always ready to teach, to open the door when we knock, and to be found when we seek Him (Jer 29:13; Luke 1:9–10).

---

[9] Frank Sheed, *The Church and I* (Garden City, NY: Doubleday, 1974), 238.

As Pope John Paul II's Theology of the Body teaches us, Jesus is not an abstract Savior. He is most accessible. Solid. You can throw your arms around Him. At the Last Supper, Jesus did not say, "This is my soul," or, "This is my spirit," or, "This is my teaching." He said, "This is my body—which is given up for you" (see Luke 22:19). He saved us in and through His body and we ultimately join Him in and through ours. Our sexual identities as men and women are swept up into His bodily redemption and made whole.

So the teaching of *Humanae Vitae* is not proposed in a vacuum, isolated from the whole body of Catholic sexual ethics, which itself may be likened to the popular game Jenga. The game begins with a tower built of levels of slender wooden blocks, three blocks per level. The object is to remove a block from an established level and place it on top of the tower without toppling the whole structure. The tower becomes increasingly unstable and eventually topples. You never know if you've taken out a vital block until it's too late. *Humanae Vitae*, with its insistence that sex always retain its natural ordination to new human life, is like a wooden peg at the bottom of the tower. It looks small and out-of-the-way, but remove it and the whole structure comes apart. If it stays where it is, the tower remains standing strong. It's the key-peg, so to speak.

In other words, if *Humanae Vitae* is right, then all other uses of the sexual instinct that are shorn from its natural connection with conception—masturbation, sodomy, adultery and fornication, bestiality, and the like—are wrong. But if the encyclical is wrong, on what grounds and with what consistency do we argue against any of these other behaviors? The norms taught in the encyclical, and the whole body of Christian teaching on sex that precede and complement it, have as their most basic building block the idea that intercourse should never be unnaturally robbed of its procreative potential.

This book was written primarily for practicing Catholics, although Evangelicals and other believers in Christ may wish to discover the depth of the biblical roots that support the ancient Christian rejection of contraception. A growing number of Protestants are coming to appreciate the "Catholic position"—itself a misnomer insofar as it was the position of all of Christendom, as we will see, until ninety years ago. In theory, all human beings, regardless of religion, have a stake in the teaching since all of us gained our existence through the sexual embrace.[10] Even the most rabid dissenter admits of one exception to his dissent: the occasion of his own conception!

A Word about Misnomers

A few words about words. First, the word "contraception" is the most accurate term for what we are talking about. Its Latin origins capture the idea: "against the beginning," in this case, against the beginning of a new human person. Second, the term "artificial birth control" is another misnomer. The Church does not condemn birth control on the basis of artificiality (i.e., the artificial hormones of the anovulant pill or the artificial material of the condom) as opposed to "natural" methods of natural family planning, or NFP. Obviously, even the thermometer used in some methods of NFP is "artificial." At best, adding artificial as an adjective is redundant. At worst, it's misleading as to why the practice is wrong.

Further, sometimes Catholic moral theology uses technical language that can mislead the average reader. A good

---

[10] Leaving aside, for the moment, the tiny minority conceived through *in vitro* fertilization.

example is the word "evil," which conjures up images of red grinning devils brandishing pitchforks. Evil also carries the connotation that the person acting wrongly actually is evil, unless you differentiate the two. To describe an act as evil may lead some to feel qualified to judge the persons involved. That is the last impression I wish to convey. Evil simply refers to anything in which a good should exist but does not. Evil refers to a lack of a due good. It's not a substance, not a blob of badness floating around somewhere. Even Satan is good insofar as he exists. So when you see the word "evil" in these pages, think "wrong" or "immoral," not demonic or devilish.

• • •

In Chapter One, we will review the historical context that paved the way for the widespread rejection of *Humanae Vitae* and explore some reasons why it has yet to receive a fair hearing and what can be done about it. Chapter Two describes the events that brought me gradually from disagreeing altogether with the teaching, to not hating it, all the way to passionate agreement with it. If this slow-learning skeptic can defeat his doubts, anyone can.

Continuing on, the debate over birth control has jumped the fence into a much bigger field. This debate is really over who gets to decide what the will of Christ is for sex and marriage, and why. Chapter Three takes up the question, "How does God reveal Himself and what role does the Church play in communicating His Revelation?"

Chapter Four catalogues the norms of *Humanae Vitae* in the Bible. Contrary to the popular assumption that the Bible has nothing to say about birth control, God's Word consistently reverences fertility as a great gift, lauds children as blessings, and nowhere condones thwarting His gifts. Chapter Five looks at contraception in light of the Blessed Trinity and aims to show that the completely Other-directed love shared by the Father, the Son, and the Holy Spirit presents an ideal to be imitated by Christian couples and contains an implicit rejection of contraception.

Chapter Six explores the concept of natural law and how it applies to contraception. This is the philosophical heart of the book, as the Church has traditionally not invoked the Bible but the natural law to ground her opposition to contraception. Chapter Seven reveals . . . the answers to the pop quiz above.

Chapter Eight tackles an issue that comes up in many discussions about birth control, and that is the so-called "population explosion." The realities surrounding this idea verify that truth is stranger than fiction. Not only is there no population explosion, but the developed countries of the world (and many in the Third World) are now confronting a population implosion that has the real potential to cause disastrous scenarios for future generations.

Chapter Nine takes up the most popular form of contraception: sterilization. Whether it's vasectomy (male) or tubal ligation (female), both versions of the procedure entail delicate medical and pastoral challenges. It is a sensitive topic, deserving separate treatment.

Chapter Ten treats the flip side of *Humanae Vitae's* message: the "no sex without babies" principle is tied to its corollary, "no babies without sex." This edition is supplemented with new information as to why technological solutions to human problems are not always workable or even appropriate. The increased popularity of in vitro fertilization (IVF) and methods of donor insemination have brought new legal complications regarding parental rights, all of which showcases some of the unforeseen consequences of violating God's plan for sexual union.

For those who find it inconsistent that the Church condemns artificial birth control (ABC) while she promotes natural family planning (NFP), Chapter Eleven highlights the moral differences. The inability (or unwillingness) to grasp the differences between the two has proven to be a huge stumbling block for people who are trying to understand the teaching.

Chapter 12 is a brief Epilogue that explores strategies for shedding light on an issue notorious for its heat. How does the teaching work itself out in the marriage relationship? In what sense does the future belong to ambassadors of its message? Can a future Pope or Synod contradict it?

Finally, the Appendix is a list of resources for those interested in additional practical help, either in learning more about the foundations of *Humanae Vitae* and their relation to marriage, finding a good NFP-only physician, or locating a Catholic-friendly organization that provides solid educational and pastoral information.

Most Catholics who choose contraception generally do so without much investigation beyond a visit to the family doctor. Often, a kindly priest has blessed the decision or guided them along a path that can, unfortunately, lead either to a dead end or off a cliff. These couples deserve honest, loving dialogue, not finger-pointing. Liberals stress that God is love; conservatives, that God is truth. Both are half-right. The appearance of Our Lord Jesus Christ reveals that God is both love and truth (John 1:14).

Let contracepting couples, therefore, and those who would share with them the fullness of Christian teaching remember that God is a just and merciful Father and that bashing with truth is as bad as excusing with love.

Chapter One

HOW WE GOT HERE

And if the bugle gives an indistinct sound, who will get ready for battle?

—1 Corinthians 14:8

How did we get here? How did the cultural ethos change so radically from the early 1960s, and how did it reverberate so powerfully within the Catholic Church? While polling data is not always perfectly reliable, one universally accepted truth is that a majority of today's Catholics "have a problem with" the Church's teaching against contraception. Anecdotal evidence suggests it's somewhere near 90 percent, perhaps higher.

It was not always so. Among the laity and established theologians alike, there was a firm consensus until the mid-1960s that the condemnation of artificial birth control was a closed, settled issue.[1] Even those who later abandoned the ancient position of the Church and became well-known as vocal dissenters were, in the early sixties, solidly commit-

---

[1] For a succinct summary of the early controversies, see Janet E. Smith, *Humanae Vitae: A Generation Later* (Washington, DC: Catholic University of America Press, 1991), 7–18.

ted to Catholic orthodoxy on this issue. These include Karl Rahner, SJ; Fr. Andrew Greeley; Richard McCormick, SJ; Josef Fuchs, SJ; and others.

Flawed Expectations

A softening of the ground began while the sessions of the Second Vatican Council were still going on. The final draft of the Pastoral Constitution on the Church in the Modern World (known in its Latin title *Gaudium et Spes*)[2] addressed the topic of birth control but did not make any direct, explicit pronouncement since the Papal Commission on Birth begun by Pope John XIII—and enlarged by Paul VI in 1964—was still in session.[3] It is odd that a more forceful statement wasn't made in the sections dealing with marriage and family. Leftists could, and did, view the tentative tone as something of a loophole or at least a sign of things to come.

When the Council closed on December 8, 1965, the fathers had no plans to publish a definitive account regarding doctrine on birth control. The activists were meanwhile hard at work behind the scenes under the *de facto* leadership of Fr. Charles Curran—who would later play a starring role in the drama of dissent when the definitive account *did* arrive—in the sweltering summer of 1968.

---

[2] Second Vatican Council, Pastoral Constitution on the Church in the Modern World *Gaudium et Spes* (December 7, 1965), § 51 (hereafter cited in text as *GS*).

[3] Footnote fourteen reads, "Certain questions which need further and more careful investigation have been handed over, at the command of the Supreme Pontiff, to a commission for the study of population, family, and births, in order that, after it fulfills its function, the Supreme Pontiff may pass judgment. With the doctrine of the magisterium in this state, this holy synod does not intend to propose immediately concrete solutions." This is no endorsement of dissent, but seems to convey a sense of tentativeness.

The dissenters were patient, methodical, and media savvy.[4] Some claimed that the dramatic abandonment of, or silence towards, a commonly held doctrine was somehow the voice of the Holy Spirit speaking through the "voice of the laity," or the much vaunted *sensus fidelium* (sense of the faithful). They just forgot that it pertained to the faithful, not the faithless (or faith-confused).

The short answer to this is to repeat that the Catholic Church is not a democracy. If it were, then the Church of Christ would have spun itself into the Church of Arius in the fourth century, since a large majority of the faithful held to the Arian heresy.[5] What is more, in the face of bad polling numbers, Jesus would have backed down from His teaching about the Real Presence in the Eucharist.[6] Ironically, groups dissenting on contraception were led and organized primarily by clergy, including some bishops. Arguably, the strongest voices of support for Pope Paul VI have come from the laity, a sterling example being H. Lyman Stebbins, who founded Catholics United for the Faith in 1968 during the maelstrom over *Humanae Vitae* "to support the efforts of the teaching Church" as its literature proclaims.

Americans are especially enamored with the ideals of democracy. The habit of making vital decisions by a vote

---

[4] George A. Kelly examines the major players who led, and were led by, this sudden shift in "The Bitter Pill the Catholic Community Swallowed," in *Human Sexuality: What the Church Teaches Today* (Jamaica Plain, MA: Daughters of Saint Paul, 1979), 13–101.

[5] Arius (died AD 336) taught that since Jesus is the Son of God, He must be younger somehow, and therefore not truly divine. The Church's denunciation of Arianism in the Council of Nicea in AD 325 led indirectly to the development of the Nicene Creed.

[6] "After this many of his disciples drew back and no longer went about with him. Jesus said to the twelve, 'Will you also go away?' Simon Peter answered him, 'Lord, to whom shall we go? You have the words of eternal life; and we have believed, and have come to know, that you are the Holy One of God'" (John 6:66–69).

runs deep in American life. We vote on civic laws, police chiefs, mayors, presidents. On television, we vote off survivors from islands and idols off stages. And yet, as we'll see in Chapter Three, the Church was established by the authority of the Lord Jesus, not by the consent of His disciples. Jesus is Lord, on His terms. And if He is not Lord of our sexuality, He is Lord of nothing. The Church is a Bride with a Bridegroom, a Body with a Head. And her doctrines come from Him, not from a show of hands.

The shifts of the tectonic plates of culture in the direction of dissent are easy enough to track. The timing of Paul's encyclical could hardly have been worse, having appeared during the pause between the Summer of Love and the Woodstock Music Festival. "This is the dawning of the Age of Aquarius," sang the chorus in *Hair!*, the nudist musical of the day. The zeitgeist bristled with the anti-establishment ideals of Haight-Ashbury Hippies, LSD experimentation, flower children, hand-painted Volkswagen vans, "free love," and campus unrest.

For social upheaval and violence, the year 1968 was quite the year. That was the year of the Tet Offensive in Vietnam in which the Vietcong in the North surprised American and South Korean forces with massive attacks. As the Vietnam War dragged on, antiwar protests—many turning violent—spiked across the country. It was the year of the brutal My Lai Massacre in which US Army soldiers went on a killing and raping spree against unarmed civilians. Martin Luther King, Jr., and Bobby Kennedy were murdered that year, the same year the French government was almost toppled by strikes and the May student uprising. In Derry (Northern Ireland), police baton civil rights demonstrators were igniting the Troubles.

In Hollywood, the decades-old Hays Production Code was replaced with the Motion Picture Association of America (MPAA) ratings system in November of 1968.[7] Tumult was the theme, change the constant. The English historian Paul Johnson called it the year of "America's suicide attempt."[8]

Into this galloping river *Humanae Vitae* was dropped, to whirl bravely upstream like a gawky, determined salmon. And whirl it did, even though, from a worldly point of view, it carried the wrong message at the wrong time to the wrong audience.

The Catholic flock of the late 1960s was disoriented as to what was expected of them in the wake of the Second Vatican Council. Tens of thousands of priests and religious had fled their vows. As the Church recalibrated her relationship to the world, many Catholics recalibrated their relationship to the Church. Latin was everywhere eclipsed, quite against the mandates of the Council. Theological outlooks became congealed: the Right wanted only continuity with the past; the Left, with the future. For many of the ordinary faithful, the idea that conscience trumps truth had a seductive ring

---

[7] See Patrick Coffin, "Code Blue: Hollywood and Self-Censorship," in *Saint Austin Review,* vol. 2, October, 2001. Films that earned Oscar nominations from 1965 to 1973 reflect a decidedly permissive shift in the moral content of American cinema: from *A Man for All Seasons* and *The Sound of Music* to the R-rated *Midnight Cowboy* and the X-rated *Last Tango In Paris* in less than eight years. Named for a 1920s Postmaster General, the Hays Code was a set of self-imposed censorship guidelines for studios that governed the moral content of American cinema from 1934–1965. Later known as the Breen Office, named for a feisty Catholic layman named Joseph Breen, the Code was closely affiliated with the Catholic Legion of Decency, which was praised by Pius XI in the first papal encyclical on the media, *Vigilanti Cura* (1936).

[8] Cited by James Cardinal Francis Stafford in his lucid personal recollection "The Year of the Peirasmòs: 1968," originally published in *L'Osservatore Romano* on July 26, 2008, accessed at http://www.calcatholic.com/news/newsArticle.aspx?id=2782389d-da2c-40ce-8d7f-071d2345291c.

to it—an idea that would have consequences for the birth control debate, particularly in the Canada of my childhood, as we'll see in the next chapter.

Candor requires the admission that too few ecclesial leaders wanted to touch the new hot potato that bounced out of Rome, let alone impose canonical penalties for priests who rejected it publicly. What Chesterton referred to in the 1920s as "the strange mental confusion" that surrounded contraception has come back as a whirlwind of strangeness and confusion. What would G. K. think of hardcore porn available for children's viewing a click away, or the divorce rate, or the unlimited abortion license, or the transgender-mania that has gripped popular culture?

Everybody Loves a Majority

Catholics believe that popes, when they teach in union with the bishops of the world, do so infallibly in matters of faith and morals—including the common teaching of Ecumenical Councils. Again, not necessarily in temporal affairs. We can retain filial respect for leaders in the Church while affirming that not all administrative or disciplinary decisions are created equal; some have unintended and unforeseen results.

A few examples:

While the purpose of the expanded Papal Commission has never been made clear, as it grew under Paul VI's watchful eye, some of its members became virtual celebrities when portions of their deliberations were leaked to the press in 1966. Blood was in the water. Most among the vaunted Commission voted for change. Four years of whisper campaigns and fawning media coverage of the Commission's (selectively) confidential activities were never far from the news wires.

While no one believes Paul VI was a closet dissenter who finally buckled under "curial pressure," there is some evidence that he wanted the most coherent possible answer to the question, since the first birth control pill, Enovid, was given FDA approval in 1960. The late professor Germain Grisez assisted John Ford, SJ, an original member of the Commission who stood with the Church. "[Pope] Paul also thought there might be something about the Pill that was different," Grisez told an interviewer in 2003. "And, if there was, he wanted to find out about it, because he felt the Church couldn't ask something that God doesn't require of them."[9]

While widely respected, and known to be a man of deep holiness, Paul VI did not elicit the kind of spontaneous affection from the public that Pope John XXIII did with his ample girth and cherubic grin. Nor did he command the august bearing of a Pius XI or a Pius XII, neither of whom had any known allergies to confrontation. Pope Paul's work of overseeing three quarters of the Second Vatican Council got him labeled "too conservative" for the progressives and "too progressive" for the old guard. By temperament, Paul VI was more Prince Hamlet than King Lear.

Agitation for change came drop by drop, editorial by editorial. Pope Paul continued to wrestle with his response. In a private meeting with Archbishop Fulton Sheen, the Pope confided to the famous US prelate that when he (Paul VI) rested his head on his pillow at night, he felt as though it were made of thorns.[10] During his General Audience on July

---

[9] Interview with Dr. Germain Grisez by Ann Carey in "How Dissenters Tried to Sway the Birth Control Teaching," in *Our Sunday Visitor*, August 3, 2003, accessed at http://www.osvpublishing.com.periodicals/show-article.asp?pid=830. Grisez worked with John Ford, SJ, who served on the Papal Commission.

[10] Archbishop Fulton J. Sheen, *The Heart of a Pope*, taped homily, Saint Agnes Church, 1979, courtesy Ministro-Media.

31, 1968, at the end of his four-year study period, Paul VI admitted that he "trembled before alternatives," and never felt the burden of his high office more keenly in his entire papacy.

Bad Opening Night

The Commission's Majority Report, as it's colloquially known, argued for a change in the two-thousand-year-old teaching. The arguments are similar to that of the Anglican Lambeth Conference in 1930. It was almost the Hippies revisited by the Flappers. Both groups, the old Anglican bishops and the new Catholic scholars, took pains to insist that birth control is to be used only in exceptional cases— and only in marriage—so that its use would not, should not, could not, lead to any social problems like promiscuity or marital breakdown.[11]

Two years went by after the leak. Pope Paul continued to deliberate, bombarded by unremitting pressure to capitulate to the whisper of the world to consider the Pill morally neutral or even good.

When the encyclical was finally released on July 25, 1968, Paul VI inexplicably chose Monsignor Ferdinando Lambruschini to announce it at a press conference. A moral theologian at Lateran University, Monsignor Lambruschini voted for change at the final meeting of the Papal Commission.[12] During the press conference, he promptly opined

---

[11] As published in Robert McClory, *Turning Point: The Inside Story of the Papal Birth Control Commission and How* Humanae Vitae C*hanged the Life of Patty Crowley and the Future of the Chu*rch (New York, NY: Crossroad, 1995), 171–87.

[12] McClory, *Turning Point*, 138. McClory's one-sided account is relentlessly sympathetic to the part of dissent.

that the encyclical was "not infallible," and his subsequent caveats did little to undo the conclusions drawn by the press.

Never in history has a papal document of thirty-one succinct paragraphs set off such a maelstrom. The print on the paper was still warm when a protest, akin to those of Vietnam War, was organized by Fr. Charles Curran on the steps of Catholic University in Washington, DC, to denounce it. Well-organized theological elites in America issued statements and signature rolls dismissing the encyclical, which was even lampooned on TV's *Laugh-In*.

Why so short an encyclical should take so long to write may never be known. An unnamed cardinal once confided to apologist Frank Sheed that some of the Pope's advisors insisted that the first version was "held to be too long for the public's reading habits: a document half as long would be more likely to be read," Sheed recalled in his autobiography. "But instead of being rewritten at the new length, it was chopped about till it was short enough. Even on a Cardinal's word I find this hard to credit. But it would certainly explain the result."[13]

The actual encyclical, while faithfully communicating the truth about sexuality and marriage, does not argue its case so much as re-present established teaching. Professor J. Budziszewski voices this quibble while yet endorsing Paul's conclusion. In fact, Professor Budziszewski and his wife entered the Catholic Church a few years after writing these lines:

> Though addressed not only to Roman Catholics but to "all men of good will," *Humanae Vitae* is both diffuse and elliptical; its premises are scattered and,

---

[13] Sheed, *The Church and I*, 243.

to non-Catholics, obscure. Though the encyclical letter is magisterial in the sense of being lordly, it is not magisterial in the sense of teaching well. It seems to lack the sense, which any discussion of natural law requires, of what must be done to make the self-evident evident, to make the intuitive available to intuition, to make what is plain in itself plain to us.[14]

The End of the Ends?

Neither Vatican II (in *Gaudium et Spes*) nor *Humanae Vitae* employed the traditional language of Catholic sexual morality whereby procreation was seen as the primary end or purpose of sex, and the unity and pleasure as secondary ends. From this shift in approach, liberal and traditionalist critics of *Humanae Vitae* concluded that the old distinctions had been abandoned in favor of the new paradigm of the "inseparability of the procreative and the unitive meanings."[15]

But this is not the case. The linguistic shift occurred, among other reasons, to better identify with the massive, almost overnight, changes in cultural attitudes toward sexuality. A more personalist mode of communication stemmed from a new emphasis in Catholic sexual ethics whereby subjectivity—the human person and his experience of himself as man or woman—is taken as a starting point instead of objective moral norms or "rules." One could say that the entire corpus of Karol Wojtyla's writings comprise a bridge

---

[14] J. Budziszewski in "Contraception: A Symposium," in *First Things*, December 1998, 18–19.
[15] Pope John Paul II, Encyclical letter on the Regulation of Birth *Humanae Vitae* (July 25, 1968), § 12 (hereafter cited in text as HV).

between the older "manualist" approach (which is still valid) and the post-Conciliar emphasis on inner experience.[16]

Where the wording of *Casti Connubii* lays emphasis on the vertical, objective demands of God's law, *Humanae Vitae* and subsequent magisterial teaching stresses the horizontal, subjective experience of being human as a way of discovering and embracing this law. When Paul VI taught that man must not separate the procreative from the unitive meaning, he was teaching exactly what previous popes taught, albeit from another angle. Catholic teaching still affirms procreation as the primary end of sex but this does not mean that couples must always deliberately intend each sexual act to be fecund nor that the "secondary ends" of unity and pleasure are somehow unimportant.

The older approach may be harmonized with the new by seeing them as two beams, one standing vertically, the other lying horizontally. The two intersect, like the cross, the sign of contradiction par excellence.

False God Rising

Catholics have always believed that the doctrines of the Faith aren't dependent on particular ways of explaining them, nor on positive polling data. If *Humanae Vitae* bears the whiff of divine truth, it is because God has guaranteed by the Holy Spirit that the teaching is His. But other problems have appeared, which stand as a threat to accepting the teaching. One is worth singling out.

In the decades since the appearance of *Humanae Vitae*, a false god has arisen that poses a tremendous challenge to

---

[16] For a concise overview of this shift, see John S. Grabowski, *Sex and Virtue: An Introduction to Sexual Ethics* (Washington, DC: Catholic University Press, 2003).

those wishing to understand—let alone practice—the historic Christian teaching on artificial birth control. This false god's popularity shows every sign of spreading. A whole parallel religion has been thrown up in its support and in the spread of devotion to it. It has a clergy (Hugh Hefner and Larry Flynt, *et al.*), sacraments (pornography, fornication, adultery), a special rite of absolution (abortion), a devotional practice (masturbation), a creed (the Playboy philosophy), and even an evangelical revival (the Sexual Revolution).

What is it?

It is the sterilized orgasm.

As false idols go, it makes a kind of diabolical sense. If you were Satan and you wanted to draw people away from the Lord of Life, what better way to bait them than with a plausible counterfeit? Since every normal person past puberty desires sex, it's a stroke of genius to put into his or her mind that the spark of life is identical to the Flame. The false god in question doesn't steer the car off the cliff right away. That would get noticed! Rather, it deftly interferes with the car's GPS directions by providing a realistic looking substitute. Remove fertility as an organic element of orgasm, particularly the male variety, and attachment to the experience becomes instantly more likely. Turning the metaphor inside out, would Bonnie and Clyde be more likely, or less likely, to rob banks if you take away the police?

With love replaced by lust, the replacement was anointed as the equivalent of "all-sufficient grace" in this cult of the sterilized orgasm. As long as the natural tie between sex and babies remains severed, the cult can flourish. If chastity intrudes, the cult of the false god dies. Nothing like the imagined sound of a baby crying to spoil the picnic.

Snapping the Stronghold

My former spiritual director Fr. John McGoey was a kindred spirit of Servant of God Dorothy Day—she even mentions him in her autobiography, *The Long Loneliness*. This Scarboro Missionary of China wrote over a dozen books on family life and sexual maturity. One of the many McGoeyisms that have stuck with me is this: *There is nothing good about pleasure; it's merely enjoyable. And there is nothing bad about pain; it's merely unpleasant.* How many sexual and relational problems would be solved overnight if this were understood?

McGoey, who died in 1995 (I was a pallbearer at his funeral), understood well that chastity is vital to personal happiness. Chastity is to personal love, he liked to say, what budgeting is to finance. One net result of contraception has been a lowering of respect for—even the need for—the virtue of chastity. The very term "making love" suggests that love can be manufactured by sex. The truth is that only life can be made; love must be willed. Sex is no more inherently loving than a salute is inherently respectful (a soldier may despise the officer he salutes).

You can guess where this is going: Without contraception and the eclipse of chastity it provoked, the Sexual Revolution would never have gotten out of first gear. Without the ease and short-term convenience of the Pill, the Sexual Revolution would have been a Ferrari with an empty tank.

Scripturally, the inability to distinguish sex from love—which is to say the immaturity that refuses to embrace necessary pains and avoid destructive pleasures—is known as a stronghold (2 Cor 10:4). The only sure victory over a stronghold or attachment to the idol of false sexuality is a corresponding surrender to the love of the true Father. From this surrender comes victory over all created things (addictions, people, vainglory, temptations, and false idols) that prevent us from loving God aright, and our neighbor as ourselves.

Apart from commenting from time to time on the negative reaction to his encyclical, Pope Paul did not vigorously defend it. The only other major work he produced after that was the 1975 Apostolic Exhortation on Evangelization, *Evangelii Nuntiandi*. The aging Holy Father was up against a battery of resistance on all fronts in the Church as he tried to implement the norms of an Ecumenical Council in a time of profound upheaval and sexual insanity. It wasn't until Pope John Paul II made the teaching the cornerstone of his papacy that the message of *Humanae Vitae* got its groove back and, with that groove, a new chance at acceptance.

Acceptance tends to be related to one's view of authority, which, in turn, can be tied to a general crisis of faith. This was certainly true for me before my escape from dissent.

Chapter Two

ESCAPE FROM DISSENT

Is my gloom after all, Shade of His hand outstretched caressingly?

—Francis Thompson
The Hound of Heaven

In the halcyon days of my dissent, I had no real arguments against this teaching of the Church. What I had was an attitude.

I didn't *like* it.

In most respects my Catholic upbringing was typical. While Nova Scotia had no parochial school system, my public school education included weekly catechism classes and my Sundays included Mass with my father. My mother entered the Church twenty years after getting married, having been instructed by then Msgr. Colin Campbell (now-deceased bishop of Antigonish). The Catholic charismatic renewal and the Cursillo Movement swept through Eastern Canada in the late 1970s, and with them came many spiritual blessings to the local Church and to our family.

But I was a more rambunctious kid than most, and rather less teachable. I dimly recall, and my father delights to tell, one revealing anecdote. During one Sunday Mass, as the procession made its way past our pew, my dad tried to settle my five-year-old self down by pointing to the priest. Catching sight of his cape-like vestments, I supplied amusement for the congregation and mortification for my father by hollering, "Look, Dad, Batmaaaan!"

But when it came for the Consecration, I remember feeling a strange sort of awe. Though I was too young to know why, I took the light aroma of incense as a token of something entirely "other" going on in that sacred moment. I was nowhere near able to understand transubstantiation, but I somehow knew that, in the hushed moment after the shimmering bells' sound had quieted, God was *there*.

Seeds on Rocky Ground

My uncle, a permanent deacon, got a bunch of us involved in various youth events. A major turning point was a Teen Challenge retreat weekend (the youth wing of Cursillo) in which God gave me the grace of faith in Jesus Christ as God's personalized invitation to be in a relationship with Him. And I immediately wanted to know more about the Church, which had provided this life-changing experience, and to get my hands on as much theology as I could.

A bachelor's degree in religious studies and philosophy seemed like a good start. So I enrolled at the local Catholic institution of higher learning, Mount Saint Vincent University in Halifax, which still stands watch over the blue-grey Bedford Basin.

By the time I got there in the early 80s, "the Mount" had already begun to drift from its Roman Catholic moorings, institutionally beguiled by the elusive ghost known as the spirit of Vatican II. My theology syllabus read like a Who's

Who of Catholic dissenters. We got regular samplings of Hans Kung (whose lecture in Halifax was regarded by the local liberals as an Elvis appearance); ex-Dominican and now ex-Catholic Matthew Fox; ex-Augustinian Gregory Baum, who had been a *peritus* (expert advisor) at the Second Vatican Council; Richard McCormick, SJ; Bernard Häring, CSsR; Rosemary Ruether-Radford; and Fr. Richard McBrien. Even radical lesbian and self-described witch Mary Daly lectured us.[1] All of these either reject certain aspects of moral theology, have been formally censured by the magisterium, or have left their religious vows (or the Church) altogether.

It was fairly drilled into us that theologians functioned as a kind of parallel or second magisterium, and we were taught to see them as prophets speaking truth to power.[2] The fact that most of the above leaders had been in trouble with The Official Church made them all the more fashionable. These graying sages weren't going to be the Pope's automatons. They were scholars, *with PhDs and everything*.

What mattered, especially to the young and impressionable like the present writer, was that it was all so terribly cutting-edge. Better to sprint with the trail-blazers than to stumble with the papists who, by comparison, could only spout catechisms by rote. What are you going to go with, the Armani or the polyester?

This is not to pick on the Mount. Scores of Catholic universities have sold their souls since 1965. The slide of such

---

[1] Even for liberal sympathizers, the late Ms. Daly's profanity-laced appearance was astonishing. She kept to her custom of refusing to answer questions from males. Men were instructed bluntly to pass on any question we might have to a nearby woman in the crowd and she (Daly) would answer her, not the man asking the question.

[2] The term "parallel magisterium" was coined by Richard McCormick, SJ, after whom a public lecture series was named at Mount Saint Vincent.

colleges into secularity has been well documented in *The Dying of the Light* by Fr. James Burtchaell, CSC, and *The Soul of the American University* by George Marsden, and in the experience of anyone who was an adult at the close of Vatican II. In fairness, my professors were dedicated, friendly, and gifted. I don't remember anyone setting out to offend, and I admired them as teachers and Christian educators. Put charitably, however, a commitment to Catholic orthodoxy was not an institutional priority.

Stripped of academes, the gist was that one's commitment to Christ could bypass the Church's magisterium depending on how much of a "problem" you had with a given teaching and on how much you "prayerfully considered your choices." That was pretty much the criteria. (See the Winnipeg Statement later in this chapter.) The Church was assumed to be standing between God and us, as opposed to sacramentally uniting us with Him—the classic Protestant objection to Catholicism.

A key presupposition here was that Church doctrine could change from one era to the next and that a "plurality" (liberal code for "contradictory") of theological opinion was not merely inevitable or worrisome—it was marvelous. Integral to my reversion to the Faith was the discovery that doctrine develops organically, like a cub into a lion, not a kitten into a warthog. Christ's doctrine grows richer over time without fragmenting into clashing viewpoints. In other words, while it can be expanded and deepened, Christian teaching in one generation can't be contradicted in the next.

While the Catholic Church recognizes the legitimacy of withholding public assent if a given doctrine is in doubt—a rare occurrence in itself, and pertaining mainly to professional theologians—what I signed onto was beyond that. In waving the flag of dissent, and doing my best to ignore the inconsistency, I'd crossed some mysterious mental line. It's embarrassing to recall how long it took me to see that "disagree" and "faithful" are mutually exclusive.

The Gospel according to Jiminy Cricket

Powering the engine of dissent is a popular, and mistaken, view of conscience. The Second Vatican Council, in the document *Gaudium et Spes* ("The Pastoral Constitution on the Church in the Modern World") indeed taught the importance of conscience:

> Deep within his conscience man discovers a law that he has not laid upon himself but which he must obey. Its voice, ever calling him to love and do what is good and to avoid evil, tells him inwardly at the right moment: do this, shun that. For man has in his heart a law inscribed by God. His dignity lies in observing this law, and by it he will be judged. His conscience is man's most secret core, and his sanctuary. There he is alone with God whose voice echoes in his depths. (16)

These sensible words were twisted to mean that one may pick and choose among doctrines because, well, we can veer safely from "the pope's teaching" because his is only one Christian voice among many—although we must "take it respectfully into account." As theologian Jiminy Cricket said to layman Pinocchio, "Let your conscience be your guide."

Protestants could keep *Sola Scriptura* (by Scripture alone) and *Sola Fide* (by Faith alone); we had *Sola Consciencia* (by Conscience alone).

At least in Canada, by far the most influential post–

Vatican II document on the matter of conscience relative to birth control appeared eight weeks after *Humanae Vitae* was issued. It was the Canadian bishops' response to *Humanae Vitae*, dubbed the "Winnipeg Statement" after the Manitoba city where they met. Most Catholics wouldn't recognize the Winnipeg Statement if it was posted on their fridges in neon. But as a symbol of St. Paul's "uncertain sound" (1 Cor 14:8), its effects nonetheless echoed down the teaching arm of the Church to my native Canada, and far beyond our shores.

Being one of the very first responses from the world's episcopal conferences, it undoubtedly influenced the statements from Scandinavia, Austria, West Germany, the Netherlands, and Belgium, all of which openly tried to dilute Paul VI's absolute prohibition of contraception. As elsewhere, a popular American high school religion textbook still repeats the false claim that Pope Paul VI approved of the Statement.[3]

The document begins in harmony with the encyclical, but ends with a note of doubt so glaring that the English language editor of *L'Osservatore Romano* declined to run it.[4] "Thus in accord with the accepted principles of moral theology," announced paragraph 26, "if these persons have tried sincerely but without success to pursue a line of conduct in keeping with the given directives, they may be safely assured that, *whoever* honestly chooses that course which seems right to him does so in good conscience."

As long as he "tries sincerely" to "honestly choose" to do "what seems right to him," one does so "in good conscience"?

---

[3] Mark Link, SJ, *Path through Catholicism* (Thomas More Book Association, 1991), 204–205.

[4] See Vincent N. Foy, *Birth Control: Is Canada Out of Step with Rome?* (Toronto: Life Ethics Information Centre, 2005), 93. Also, Lambert Greenan, OP, former English-language editor, *L'Osservatore Romano*. Personal interview, March 20, 2004.

It's difficult to imagine any other Christian instruction so coiled up in caveats. Would the same kind of love-bomb phrasing be applied to, say, stealing, racism, adultery, ruining the environment, or exploiting the poor? Despite assurances from its defenders, the Winnipeg Statement was, and is, interpreted as a *de facto* license to dissent.

The final paragraph quotes Cardinal Newman: "Lead kindly light amidst the encircling gloom." Given the mixed message of the Statement and its repeated emphasis on the difficulties involved in following the Church's teaching, it's reasonable to interpret the gloom as an allusion not to the forces of secularism or temptation, but to the encyclical itself.

You can't get squeezed toothpaste back into the tube, but you can start brushing. On December 12, 1973, the Canadian Catholic Conference of Catholic Bishops (CCCB) issued a Statement on the Formation of Conscience, which, while not explicitly mentioning *l'Affair* Winnipeg, tried to shore up the flood tide by making a strong case for the authentic Catholic view of conscience.

On April 3, 1989, the bishops of Manitoba released a solid defense of the encyclical titled *Responsible Parenthood*.

On June 30, 2003, a sub-committee of the Canadian bishops known as the Catholic Organization for Life and Family (COLF) issued *The Church Says Yes to Love*, a warm commemoration of the thirty-fifth anniversary of Paul VI's encyclical.

In May, 2008, speaking at the convocation of Our Lady Seat of Wisdom Academy in Ontario, Archbishop of Ottawa Terrance Prendergast, SJ, pleasantly surprised his audience by saying,

> The encyclical gives the Church a deeper understanding into the beauty of married love and responsible

parenthood. It offers a clearer understanding of the harm of contraception and the great value of Natural Family Planning (NFP). Further, it challenges married couples, healthcare professionals and clergy to live and teach these profound truths about human sexuality and dignity.[5]

In March of 1988, the Austrian bishops retracted their problematic 1968 response to *Humanae Vitae*.[6] Hopefully, other national Conferences will, in time, follow their brother bishops' lead in amending their initial reaction. Regardless, all spiritual fathers whom God has placed over us in Christ need and deserve our prayers and encouragement. If you want to know what is expected of bishops, their high duties are found in the Vatican II document *Christus Dominus*.[7] The Church's standard for her bishops is exceedingly high, as it should be.

In September, 2008, the Canadian bishops issued a *de facto* repudiation of their Winnipeg Statement, almost exactly forty years later. It is a clarion call to fidelity to *Humanae Vitae*, a strongly worded challenge to the faithful to reexamine what it calls Pope Paul's "prophetic" teaching. It is robustly titled *Liberating Potential* and even cites the work of Christopher West, the popular exponent of John Paul II's Theology of the Body. Here is a short sample:

---

[5] As quoted in John-Henry Westen, "Archbishop: For the Clergy, Obedience to Church Requires Preaching about the Moral Evil of Contraception," *LifeSiteNews*, http://www.lifesitenews.com/ldn/2008/may/08051302.html.

[6] Vincent N. Foy, "Tragedy at Winnipeg," *Challenge Magazine*, 1988, reprinted with permission by LifeSite.net.

[7] "Decree Concerning the Pastoral Office of Bishops in the Church"; Vatican archive URL found here: http://www.vatican.va/archive/hist_councils/ii_vatican_council/documents/vat-ii_decree_19651028_christus-dominus_en.html.

Nevertheless, *Humanae Vitae* is much more than a "no to contraception." This encyclical is in reality a major reflection on God's design for human love. It proposes a vision of "the whole man and the whole mission to which he is called . . . both its natural, earthly aspects, and its supernatural, eternal aspects." It is an invitation to be open to the grandeur, beauty and dignity of the Creator's call to the vocation of marriage.[8]

This is all a great start, but given the scandal and confusion it has wrought, the Winnipeg Statement needs to be publicly corrected.

Getting Unstuck is Harder than Getting Stuck

I certainly don't blame the Winnipeg Statement alone for my recalcitrance. The theological training I received undercut the bishops as teachers in the first place. Nor do I recall holding any fancy theories that kept me from accepting *Humanae Vitae.* Only after I reverted to "full meal deal" Catholicism did I learn the philosophical principles behind most forms of dissent in the Church.

The battle over *Humanae Vitae* is connected to the much broader question of the ecclesial relationship between the governed and those who govern (and teach, and sanctify). By far, the greatest success of the parallel magisterium has been to undermine confidence in the Church's credibility to teach "bedroom zone" doctrine at all. If ordinary Catholics could be convinced that obedience to allegedly non-infallible doctrine was an open question, next up at bat would be

---

[8] See http://www.cccb.ca/site/content/view/2636/1214/lang,eng/.

fornication, homosexuality, in vitro fertilization, remarriage after divorce, and abortion—the whole cohort of what dissenters snidely call "pelvic issues."

In truth, my "problem with" *Humanae Vitae* was just an important-sounding way of saying I was confused and divided. Buying into the contraceptive mentality was of a piece with that confusion. I suffered a major blind spot that I've since found is very common: I was unable to see the difference between birth prevention through contraception and birth regulation through natural family planning, which I treat in Chapter Ten.

On the one hand, dissenters try to make the case that NFP and contraception are essentially the same thing. But if challenged to simply give NFP a try—you know, no negative side effects, an easy-to-learn method, and a high effectiveness rate—they protest, "No way, they're different!"

Exactly right. They're different, and *how*. For couples with a serious reason to postpone pregnancy, natural family planning demands a level of self-mastery that contraception never does. Yet it's possible to deny what you know.

Cardinal Newman once said that ten thousand difficulties do not make one doubt. Although there was no single thunderbolt moment, over time the desire to work through the difficulties bested the stamina of my doubts. Up to that point I doubted everything save my doubts. The closest I came to a "Eureka" was the slowly percolating idea that contraception squashes a woman's capacity for fertility, turning every day into an infertile day. Contraception is sex plus some device; NFP is sex interspersed with abstinence. More about this in Chapter Eleven.

In other words, I had to admit that abstaining from sex on a day believed to be fertile is not morally identical with engaging in it while simultaneously undercutting its life-giving power. A no to contraception implied a yes to NFP, which implied a yes to chastity, which implied self-denial, which implied good old-fashioned repentance, which implied a revolution in my whole life. Jesus Christ was telling me through His Church that contraception was a grave sin, a telling that had two thousand years of unbroken unanimity behind it.

All this made me see where the arrow would hit. And I shrank back. Changing a mind is a cinch compared to changing a will, and this is acutely true in the area of sex. The poet W. H. Auden put his finger on what ailed me: "We would rather be ruined than changed. We would rather die in our dread than climb the cross of the moment and see our illusions die."[9]

Argument *No*; Witness *Sí*

I needed to look at Pope Paul's encyclical on its own terms, not filtered through the kaleidoscope of dissenting commentators. So I did something radical.

I read it.

And what I found, or rather what I did not find, surprised me: Paul VI didn't deploy any arguments to speak of. In fact, he doesn't appear to have written it to persuade at all. Apart from setting out some basic principles, Paul VI simply reiterates the ancient teaching, albeit in language more in sync with the modern ear. (Indeed, Papal Commission appointee Archbishop Karol Wojtyla's influence is said to be in the encyclical's elliptical style and its overtures to personalism, even though the Communist government in Poland did not permit him to travel to Rome during its writing.)

---

[9] W. H. Auden, *The Age of Anxiety: A Baroque Eclogue* (London: Faber, 1948).

This non-argumentation thing intrigued me. It was as though Paul VI was simply stating, "This is the Christian tradition: every sexual act must be open to new life. Are you with Us or not?" The response is ours to make. After all, the Church hadn't offered arguments on behalf of the Resurrection either, but apostolic testimony. *Humanae Vitae* was Pope Paul's apostolic testimony, the one for which history will remember him. Though he reigned a decade more, he never wrote another encyclical.

But I had another problem. If I charged the Church with being wrong on contraception, on what basis did I trust her with being right about, say, the canon of Scripture—or about any other revealed doctrine? I could reject *Humanae Vitae* by an appeal to conscience only if there was some shakiness about the certainty of the teaching. But the shakiness was in me. The first of my dominoes of dissent began to teeter.

In the end, it was a matter of asking for the grace to begin *to begin* to be open to the teaching. That proved a decisive turning point, after which things got easier.

Very often, the timing of one's openness is as decisive as the openness itself. Within days of willing to be open to the truth, a series of articles, evangelical Catholics, books, tapes, and essays written by defenders of the Church's teaching popped up in front of me with lovely, almost comic, timing. Not just "facts" I didn't know, but new ways of seeing the coherence between the part (*Humanae Vitae*) and the whole (Catholic sexual ethics), insights into deep connections between the premise of contraception and the conclusion of abortion, and, finally, a grasp of the moral difference between natural family planning and contraception.

The first domino toppled into the next, then the next. I ran into something I'd only read about: the fresh air of Christian orthodoxy. Here was Frank Sheed, Scott Hahn, Peter Kreeft,

Thomas Howard; there was Archbishop Fulton Sheen, G. K. Chesterton, and a host of others—my own personal cloud of witnesses—tossing me a climber's rope, showing me the next foothold, encouraging me upward.

On birth control specifically, one writer swayed above the pack like a sunflower. Her name was G. E. M. Anscombe (1919–2001), an English analytical philosopher whose 1972 lecture was later printed as *Contraception and Chastity*.[10] It is a bracing trek across the landscape of marriage, human sexuality, and the role of the Church in bringing Christ's Revelation to us. Dr. Anscombe's sharp prose chiseled away at what was left of my mental flab. (That she enjoyed a cigar only added to her charm.)

She closed with this observation: "The teaching which I have rehearsed is indeed against the grain of the world, against the current of our time. But that, after all, is what the Church as teacher is for. The truths that are acceptable to a time—these will be proclaimed not only by the Church: the Church teaches also those truths that are hateful to the spirit of an age."

Dr. Anscombe had my number. Writer-blogger Kathy Shaidle clothes the same idea in Gen X garments:

> It's not called The Holy Girlfriend Church. We don't get to hold out for the green-eyed redhead of our self-centered fantasies. Mother is Mother: demanding, set in her ways, and often an embarrassment, especially when she talks about touchy topics in front of our cool friends, wears that awful old pantsuit, makes us wear a scarf. Mother says no, and your

---

[10] Elizabeth Anscombe, *Contraception and Chastity* (London: Catholic Truth Society, 1977).

Girlfriend never would. Your Girlfriend would let you change the rules in the middle of the game, so you could win. Every night would be poker night with the boys. She'd never get old and boring and senile. Or embarrassing. The Holy Girlfriend Church exists. It just isn't the Catholic one, and never will be.[11]

Fickle and ultimately apathetic Girlfriend was no match for the fierce embrace of Mother, in the way a lemming is no match for a lioness. In the end, I found that the only toll to be paid during the escape from dissent was repentance. I got a *deal*.

Many people today equate authority with authoritarianism. The next few chapters will turn to the sources of Catholic authority to see how God's Revelation is in harmony with human reason; then we'll see how these sources have treated birth control since biblical times.

---

[11] Kathy Shaidle, "so this morning I woke up thinking . . ." *Relapsed Catholic*, www.relapsedcatholic.blogspot.com, May 4, 2007 (accessed February 18, 2008).

Chapter Three

WHO'S YOUR DADDY?
Sources of Catholic Authority

About Jesus Christ and the Church, I simply know they're just one thing, and we shouldn't complicate the matter.

—St. Joan of Arc at her trial

The question "Where is *that* in the Bible?" often presupposes that the Bible is the only source of God's Revelation. But before we examine the trees (the biblical passages that underpin the Church's teaching), it's advantageous to first see the forest (the way God has revealed Himself to us).

As we said in the introduction, behind the debate over birth control lurk broader questions such as who gets to say what God has revealed, and why. We all know what Christ said. But what did He *mean*? And who says?

This chapter attempts to answer the "Who Says" question by demonstrating how God's self-communication flows from a two-fold source: Sacred Scripture and Sacred Tradition. It may seem at first far removed from our topic, but the rewards of looking at the big picture of Catholic authority are well worth it. *Humanae Vitae* did not emerge out of nowhere, but flowed from a legitimate exercise of authority given by Jesus Christ.

The central plank on which the encyclical is built is not primarily biblical, but philosophical. Still, the Bible itself supports and confirms the Church's claim to be the authentic interpreter of natural law. This interpretation, or body of teaching about the meaning and application of the Bible, dating back to apostolic times, is known as Sacred Tradition.

With a Capital "T"

When Evangelicals, Pentecostals, and other "non-denominational" Christians see the word "tradition" used in the context of religious authority, they invariably identify it with Christ's condemnation of the "traditions of men" (Mark 7:8, 13; Matt 15:3, 6–9) that "nullify God's word" and add useless practices that hinder the journey to salvation. Because they hold to *sola scriptura* (the belief that the Bible alone is the rule of faith), they conclude that any "addition" to God's written Word is superfluous and confusing at best, blasphemous and dangerous at worst.

But when the Catholic Church speaks of Tradition with a capital T, it means something entirely different. Since the time of the apostles, Catholics have understood that God has revealed Himself by way of two distinct modes of transmission: the oral transmission of the Gospel by the apostles and their successors (which came first), and the written transmission, in particular the twenty-seven books of the New Testament (which came second).[1] The entire deposit of faith

---

[1] The New Testament was not officially canonized by the Church until the Councils of Hippo (AD 393) and Carthage (AD 419), and finally "closed," i.e., ratified, by the Council of Trent in the sixteenth century.

(*depositum fidei*) given by Jesus Christ is the Sacred Tradition of which the New Testament is the written aspect.

In other words, Scripture is part of the greater Tradition. More accurately still, as popular Bible teacher Jeff Cavins observes, "Scripture *is* Tradition" (emphasis mine).[2] The Second Vatican Council summarizes their inter-relationship this way:

> Hence there exists a close connection and communication between sacred tradition and Sacred Scripture. For both of them, flowing out of the same divine well-spring, come together in some fashion to form one thing and move towards the same end. . . . Therefore both sacred tradition and Sacred Scripture are to be accepted and venerated with the same sense of loyalty and reverence.[3]

Scripture Is Tradition

When the New Testament uses the word "tradition" to denote orally transmitted truth, it is not even argued but assumed to be on equal footing with God's written Word. The following review, which borrows heavily from a useful tract published by Catholic Answers titled *Scripture and Tradition*,[4] summarizes the main positive biblical references to tradition.

---

[2] Jeff Cavins, "Scripture Is Tradition," *Envoy Magazine*, May/June 1997.
[3] Second Vatican Council, Sacred Constitution on Divine Revelation *Dei Verbum* (November 18, 1965), § 9 (hereafter cited in text as DV). See also Matthew 28:20.
[4] Catholic Answers, "Scripture and Tradition" (2004), http://www.catholic.com/library/Scripture_and_Tradition.asp (accessed January 5, 2008).

- St. Paul urges the Thessalonians to "stand firm and hold to the traditions which you were taught by us, either by word of mouth or by letter" (2 Thess 2:15).
- He writes to Timothy, "what you have heard from me before many witnesses entrust to faithful men who will be able to teach others also" (2 Tim 2:2). There is no mention here of reliance upon on anything written, since the writing of the New Testament was barely underway.
- Paul refers to what he has received from the Lord and His disciples and to what he now hands on to the believers in Corinth: "For I delivered to you as of first importance what I also received, that Christ died for our sins in accordance with the scriptures.... Whether then it was I or they, so we preach and so you believed" (1 Cor 15:3, 11).
- The apostle praises those who follow the Sacred Tradition given by him: "I commend you because you remember me in everything and maintain the traditions even as I have delivered them to you" (1 Cor 11:2). He goes so far as to hold up his own conduct as a living exemplar for the new Corinthian Christians, promptly telling them to obey his spoken, preached word: "Be imitators of me, as I am of Christ" (1 Cor 11:1).
- According to St. Peter, the Gospel of Jesus will always be taught orally: "'but the word of the Lord abides for ever.' That word is the good news which was *preached* to you" (1 Pet 1:25, emphasis mine).
- Jesus identified His own teaching with that of His apostles: "He who hears you hears me, and he who rejects you rejects me" (Luke 10:16), and He later commissioned them, not to write books, but to "Go

therefore and make disciples of all nations" (Matt 28:19). How? By preaching and teaching. For "faith comes from what is heard, and what is heard comes by the preaching of Christ" (Rom 10:17).

- The first Christians "devoted themselves to the apostles' teaching" (Acts 2:42) long before there was a New Testament. The fullness of Christian teaching was to be found not in a book but in the teaching Church, the living presence of Christ. St. Paul himself quotes a saying of Jesus that does not appear in any of the Gospels: "It is more blessed to give than to receive" (Acts 20:35). The Gospels themselves are oral tradition that has been written down.

- St. Luke opens his Gospel by stating what was derived from reliable oral testimony: "Inasmuch as many have undertaken to compile a narrative of the things which have been accomplished among us, just as they were delivered to us by those who from the beginning were eyewitnesses and ministers of the word, it seemed good to me also, having followed all things closely for some time past, to write an orderly account for you, most excellent Theophilus, that you may know the truth concerning the things of which you have been informed" (Luke 1:1–4).

- Christ did not promise that the gates of hell would not prevail against the Bible, but that they would not prevail against the Church (Matt 16:18). The New Testament itself declares *the Church* to be "the pillar and bulwark of the truth" (1 Tim 3:15).

- The truth of the faith has been given first of all to the leaders of the Church (Eph 3:5), who, with the Lord Jesus, form the foundation of the Church (Eph 2:20). The Church is guided by the Holy Spirit, who

protects the teaching of Christ from corruption and error (John 14:25–26, 16:13).
- Acts 15 describes one of the first crises of the early Church, which concerned whether new converts must be circumcised in accord with the Mosaic practice. The Old Testament obviously had no answer, and the New didn't exist yet. What then was the rightful authority that could decide? Paul and Barnabas knew. They took the question "up to Jerusalem" and asked the apostles and presbyters. After hearing Peter's negative answer, they discussed the matter and were in unanimous agreement: no requirement for circumcision. A letter was sent, which read, "We have therefore sent Judas and Silas, who themselves will tell you the same things by word of mouth. For it has seemed good to the *Holy Spirit and to us* to lay upon you no greater burden than these necessary things" (Acts 15:27–28, emphases mine), and then the letter lists some other customary prohibitions. Here are joined two key elements of Catholic authority: tradition and infallibility.

Proving Too Much

The classic verse used by Protestants to reject the validity of Sacred Tradition is 2 Timothy 3:16–17: "All Scripture is inspired by God and profitable for teaching, for reproof, for correction, and for training in righteousness, that the man of God may be complete, equipped for every good work." Enlisting Paul to refute Tradition, though, is refuted in two ways.

The first is that Paul is merely telling Timothy that Scripture is inspired and profitable for the uses he mentions (which it is!), not that it's sufficient. The second problem is summed up by the literary maxim "a text without a context is a pretext." The previous verses show that Paul is actually endorsing Sacred Tradition along with Scripture: "But as for you, continue in what you have learned and have firmly believed, knowing from whom you learned it, and how from childhood you have been acquainted with the sacred writings which are able to instruct you for salvation through faith in Christ Jesus" (2 Tim 3:14–15).

Since several other Epistles had not been written when Paul wrote to young Timothy, the "sacred writings" and "Scripture" to which he refers must be the Old Testament.

So God's Word comes to us from two closely related sources, Scripture and Tradition. But how are these concretely applied to each generation?

We Weren't "Left Behind"

Any authoritative document requires a living authority to interpret its contents. We see this clearly in the political and commercial realm. How long would a country remain stable without a Supreme Court of some kind to interpret its Constitution? How profitable would a company be without a Board of Directors to interpret its founding by-laws?

In the case of God's Word, that interpretive body is the magisterium: the pope and all bishops in union with him. Jesus our Savior is also our Teacher (*magister* is Latin for "teacher") who has "the words of eternal life" (John 6:68). He spent three or so years teaching His disciples, revealing to them the love of the Father and the way of salvation that was Himself.

But much was left untaught. Not in the sense that His teaching was less than the fullness of truth, but it was incomplete insofar as it did not, and could not, answer controverted questions that arose only later, such as: Was He truly God incarnate? If so, how? Is God a Trinity? What's the ethical status of first-strike nuclear war? Is embryonic stem cell research morally licit? In light of advanced pain-relief technology, can euthanasia be okay? How about masturbation? Or in vitro fertilization? Should infants be baptized? Ought we clone human beings?

And, more pertinent to this chapter: Which books belong in the New Testament?

Christ touched explicitly on none of these questions, yet getting the answers right is vital to being a disciple. This is especially true when it comes to the meaning of Scripture itself. Individual interpretation of what any given passage means, or does not mean, doesn't work for the simple reason that all heretics claim biblical support for their heresy. St. Peter points out the danger of the "me and my Bible" approach when he writes, "First of all you must understand this, that no prophecy of scripture is a matter of one's own interpretation" (2 Pet 1:20).

Referring to Paul's letters, Peter adds, "There are some things in them hard to understand, which the ignorant and unstable twist to their own destruction, as they do the other scriptures" (2 Pet 3:16).

Jesus did not leave us orphans. He entrusted the truths He taught—the Truth He Is—to His Church, which would be the extension of the Incarnation through time and would faithfully proclaim what her Founder taught while on earth. "Our faith in the Church is grounded in the Church's faithfulness," writes philosopher Peter Kreeft. "The Church does not have authority over Sacred Tradition because she is not its author. Its author is Christ. She can interpret it and draw out its inner meanings, but she can never correct it. She can add to it but never subtract from it; and when she adds, she adds from within, organically, as a tree adds fruit, not mechanically, as a construction crew adds another story to a house."[5]

Leaving His earthly mission unfinished, the Lord Jesus entrusted the deposit of faith to His representatives (preeminently the pope and bishops) who would spread the Gospel and "make disciples of all nations," relying all the while on the Lord's promised presence (Matt 28:19; see also John 14–17). Instituted by Christ, the organic structure of the deposit of faith is composed of Scripture, Tradition, and the magisterium.

The Second Vatican Council clarified the proper relationship between the three:

> But the task of authentically interpreting the word of God, whether written or handed on, has been entrusted exclusively to the living teaching office of the Church, whose authority is exercised in the name of Jesus Christ. This teaching office is not above the word of God, but serves it, teaching only what has been handed on, listening to it devoutly, guarding it scrupulously and explaining it faithfully in accord with a divine commission and with the help of the Holy Spirit, it draws from this one deposit of faith everything which it presents for belief as divinely revealed. (DV 10)

A simple analogy might be a great king who commissions a troubadour to write a song about the king's love for

---

[5] Peter Kreeft, *Catholic Christianity: A Complete Catechism of Catholic Belief Based on the Catechism of the Catholic Church* (San Francisco, CA: Ignatius Press, 2001), 102.

his subjects, to be sung for generations. The correct notes put down in musical notation by the troubadour correspond to the written Word of God. The actual performance of the song—lifting inert black notes up into the beautiful thing we call a melody, and the job of handing on how to phrase the notes—corresponds to Sacred Tradition and the living magisterium through time.

We see other examples of this all the time with family customs. Most families pass on traditions, from how to celebrate birthdays, to how and when to trim the Christmas tree, to favorite vacation destinations and other tried-and-true rituals. No one in the family suddenly jumps up and demands to know where these are written down. No, such traditions are "handed down" by living moms and dads without a formal rule book.

It is with the full weight of these sources of divine Revelation that the Church condemns contraception. And now the bigger fish to fry: where in Scripture do we find this condemnation?

Chapter Four

BIRTH CONTROL IN THE BIBLE
"The Silent Word Is Pleading"

Small wonder, therefore, if Holy Writ bears witness that the Divine Majesty regards with greatest detestation this horrible crime and at times has punished it with death.

—Pius XI, *Casti Connubii* (55)

Christian proponents of birth control say that the Bible is silent on the question of birth control, and that the silence speaks volumes about God's approval.

But the devil (the metaphor be pardoned) is in the details. In the following mini-tour of Sacred Scripture, we will find not silence, but a surprisingly rowdy collection of evidence in the form of clues, premises, and attitudes—along with a direct condemnation—all of which, taken together, present an airtight case that verifies the historic Christian teaching.

While the phrase "birth control" appears nowhere in Scripture, as we saw in the previous chapter God's Word often teaches certain ideas without laying out explicit definitions. In this case, what God plants in the Bible through the inspired writers He brings to fruition in Tradition through the infallible Church. (I note, only partly in jest, that the Bible also nowhere commands us to call our leaders "Reverend" or "Doctor" either, nor does it mention any of the phrases held dear by many Christians, such as "accepting Jesus as my personal Savior," "the Incarnation," "the triune God," and other ideas.)

In the case of contraception, the Bible paints a single, unambiguous picture, which is made even clearer by the magisterium. From Genesis to Revelation, the Word of God fairly vibrates with the communication of life: imparting it, communicating it, affirming it, manifesting it.[1] Human birth is always depicted as a great good, culminating particularly in the promise of a Savior to be born (Luke 1:35). The notion that sexual intercourse ought to always be open to the transmission of new life is not so much articulated as assumed in Sacred Scripture. Every biblical reference to fertility and birth is couched as a blessing; every reference to barrenness and sterility as a curse.

The Protestant Reformers looked to the Bible alone to ground their denunciations of birth control, which they hurled more stridently than any pope.[2] The onus, therefore, is on those trying to prove the contrary, since Bible-believing Christians were united for over nineteen hundred years

---

[1] Even when God carries out the death penalty, which He does a few dozen times in Scripture, it is in the interest of protecting and valuing human life or some other good.

[2] This chapter relies in part on two books by Protestant authors: *The Bible and Birth Control*, by the late Charles D. Provan; and *A Full Quiver*, by Rick and Jan Hess. These authors do not hold Catholicism in any special affection, and interestingly, they are providentialists who reject even natural family planning as immoral. The Duggar family of TV's *19 Kids and Counting* fame identify with the Quiverfull outlook.

in the conviction that contraception is against God's law. This chapter accepts that onus.

The Bible often returns to its main theme—God's marriage proposal to the soul and the restoration of all things in Christ—a theme imparted in the language of faithfulness, fruitfulness, rebirth, kinship, adoption, covenant, filial trust, and fecundity. As John Paul the Great would put it, God's Word speaks the language of nuptial union.

Some of the following verses have been examined in other chapters; I include them here for the sake of completeness. Taken together, out of many diverse times and contexts, they speak with one voice with the message that babies are blessings and that (not discounting human cooperation) God wills them to be for their own sake.

With one exception, the following is not a list of "proof texts," but evidence of a clear and consistent moral outlook. The exception is the account of Onan, in Genesis 38, which, if a text proves a doctrine, I take to be a true proof text. But regarding the rest of the list, just as a few strands of colored silk don't make a tapestry, so one or two Bible verses are insufficient to condemn all forms of birth control.

Seen one after the other, these verses reveal how solid the foundation is for the historic Christian teaching that contraception is jarringly inconsistent with the will of God.

The *First* First Commandment: Just Do It

In the following passages, the italics are mine for emphasis. The Bible's explicitly pro-fecundity attitude appears at the very beginning, in the Book of Genesis:

> So God created man in his own image, in the image of God he created him; male and female he created

them. And God blessed them, and God said to them, "*Be fruitful and multiply*, and fill the earth and subdue it; and have dominion over the fish of the sea and over the birds of the air, and over every living thing that moves upon the earth." (Gen 1:27-28)

Notice how the very act by which children are made—the physical basis of fruitfulness and multiplication—is given as a blessing to the couple. God's first commandment is simultaneously a blessing, and is addressed to *adam* (Hebrew for mankind, male and female). This is the primordial unity to which Jesus points the Pharisees in His teaching against divorce in Matthew 19, back before sin "hardened the hearts" of lovers. Moses' allowance of divorce ("For your hardness of heart," as it states in verse 8) is contrasted negatively against the original order of things that Jesus came to restore.

Before the flood, "God blessed Noah and his sons, and said to them, '*Be fruitful and multiply,* and fill the earth'" (Gen 9:1).

Not many people know that this same commandment is repeated after the flood: "And God said to him, 'I am God Almighty: *be fruitful and multiply*; a nation and a company of nations shall come from you, and kings shall spring from you'" (Gen 35:11).

Even fewer people know about the Bible's third "Be fruitful"! The hearer in this verse is Jacob—or rather Israel, since God has just changed his name following his nocturnal wrestling match with the angel in chapter 32. Any teaching repeated by God three times should give us pause. Further, contrary to the thinking of some dissenters, these verses do not apply only to Jews, since "Jew" comes from Judah, one of the sons of Jacob who arrives after these commandments.

These divine directives (thrice repeated and never revoked) must apply to humanity, not merely to a few distant Old Testament figures.

> And all these blessings shall come upon you and overtake you, if you obey the voice of the Lord your God. Blessed shall you be in the city, and blessed shall you be in the field. *Blessed shall be the fruit of your body*, and the fruit of your ground, and the fruit of your beasts. . . . And the *Lord will make you abound in prosperity, in the fruit of your body*, and in the fruit of your cattle, and in the fruit of your ground, within the land which the Lord swore to your fathers to give you. (Deut 28:2–4, 11)

This is one of the first scriptural indications that children are divine gifts, inseparable from the other elements of God's provision and care. Here are a few more:

> Of He'man, the sons of Heman: Bukki'ah, Mattani'ah, Uz'ziel, Shebu'el and Jer'imoth, Hanani'ah, Hana'ni, Eli'athah, Giddal'ti, and Romam'ti-e'zer, Joshbeka-sh'ah, Mallo'thi, Hothir, Maha'z-ioth. And these were the sons of He'man the king's seer, according to the promise of God to exalt him; for *God had given Heman fourteen sons and three daughters*. (1 Chron 25:4–5)

This charmingly named passel of children was given to Heman by God, not to annoy, disgust, or punish him, but to exalt him. So, too, in the following chapter: "And O'bed-e'dom had sons: Shemai'ah the first-born, Jeho'zabad the second, Jo'ah the third, Sachar the fourth, Nethan'el the fifth, Am'mi-el the sixth, Is'sachar the seventh, and Pe-ul-

'lethai the eighth; *for God blessed him*" (1 Chron 26:4–5).

Psalm 127 is a classic Old Testament text on the subject: "Lo, *sons are a heritage from the Lord, the fruit of the womb a reward*. Like the arrows in the hand of a warrior are the sons of one's youth. Happy is the man who has his quiver full of them! He shall not be put to shame when he speaks with his enemies in the gate" (Ps 127:3–5).

Again we see children depicted as coming from the creative hand of God as a reward, quite the opposite of a burden. The arrows-in-a-quiver imagery is rich in connotation. A quiver was part of a soldier's ordinary equipment, a long shoulder-mounted sheath used to hold arrows. The Psalmist extols a full quiver, not a moderately loaded one. What warrior in his right mind feels great about storming into battle with only 2.1 arrows in his quiver?

Regardless of how many actual arrows the average Hebrew quiver could hold (Scripture is not here demanding that mothers become non-stop "arrow factories"), the point is that God wants us to think maximally, not minimally, about our quiver's capacity, and to remain open to the blessing of arrows He might bestow. As God Himself is called a warrior in Scripture (Jer 20:11; Zeph 3:17; Job 16:14), the arrows of our full quivers—our children and their children—are also held in His hand, for His purposes.

As we know, some couples try for many years without having children, yet without stifling their "arrow-producing" union. Others, for various medical or other reasons, can only have one or two children. "Quiverfulness" is not determined by mathematics but by genuine discernment of a couples' generosity.

"Your wife will be *like a fruitful vine* within your house; your children will be like olive shoots around your table" (Ps 128:3). Olive shoots are like arrows in that they also symbolize the future spreading outward. (Olive trees can live and bear fruit for hundreds of years.) The bounteous image of olive shoots extending *around the table* says something about our 2.1 child standard.

The True Opener and Closer of Wombs

Then Abraham prayed to God; and God healed Abim'elech, and *also healed his wife and female slaves so that they bore children.* For the Lord had closed all the wombs of the house of Abim'elech because of Sarah, Abraham's wife. (Gen 20:17–18)

When the Lord saw that Leah was hated, *he opened her womb*; but Rachel was barren. And Leah conceived and bore a son, and she called his name Reuben; for she said, "Because the Lord has looked upon my affliction; surely now my husband will love me." She conceived again and bore a son, and said, "Because the Lord has heard that I am hated, *He has given me this son* also;" and she called his name Simeon. (Gen 29:31–33)

Jacob's anger was kindled against Rachel, and he said, "Am I in the place of God, who has withheld from you the fruit of the womb?" . . . Then Rachel said, "God has judged me, and has also heard my voice and *given me a son*;" therefore she called his name Dan. . . . And God hearkened to Leah, and she conceived and bore Jacob a fifth son. Leah said, "*God has given me my hire* because I gave my maid to my husband;" so she called his name Is'sachar. . . . Then God remembered Rachel, and God hearkened to her and *opened her womb*. She conceived and bore a son, and said, "God has taken away my reproach"; and she called his name Joseph, saying, "*May the Lord add to me another son!*" (Gen 30:2, 6, 17–18, 22–24)

The Lord did indeed add another son. His name was Benjamin. Had Rachel used contraception after the birth of Joseph, our New Testament would be wafer thin. It would skip from the Acts of the Apostles to the Letters of Peter and John, and the Apocalypse. For if you take away Benjamin, you take away the Letters of St. Paul because the Apostle proudly reminds us in Romans 11:2 that he's a descendent of Benjamin!

. . . although [Elka'nah] loved Hannah, he would give Hannah only one portion, because *the Lord had closed her womb.* And her rival used to provoke her sorely, to irritate her, because the Lord had closed her womb. . . . And [Hannah] vowed a vow and said, "O Lord of hosts, if thou wilt indeed look on the affliction of thy maidservant, and remember me, and not forget thy maidservant, but wilt *give to thy maidservant a son,* then I will give him to the Lord all the days of his life, and no razor shall touch his head." (1 Sam 1:5–6, 11)

They rose early in the morning and worshiped before the Lord; then they went back to their house at Ramah. And Elka'nah knew Hannah his wife, and the Lord remembered her; and in due time Hannah conceived and bore a son, and she called his name Samuel, for she said, "*I have asked him of the Lord.*" (1 Sam 1:19–20)

Notice a pattern? Without in any way canceling out the secondary cause of human meeting and mating, God repeatedly shows Himself to be the first cause of new little persons. The penultimate source of human life is sexual relations; the ultimate source is God. The Psalms return to this idea: "Know that the Lord is God! *It is he that made us,* and we are his" (Ps 100:3).

And also:

> ... my frame was not hidden from thee, when I was being made in secret, intricately wrought in the depths of the earth. Thy eyes beheld my unformed substance; in thy book were written, every one of them, the days that were formed for me, when as yet there was none of them. How precious to me are thy thoughts, O God! (Ps 139:15–17)

We postmodern Westerners have unconsciously imbibed a Darwinian way of interpreting life events by identifying God's mysterious hidden designs with random, non-rational forces.[3] The biblical writers, however, saw no contradiction in holding simultaneously that (a) God causes human life to be, and (b) human beings cause human life to be. Look at any stage play. What the playwright ultimately wants for his characters does not, from the perspective of the play's created universe, arbitrarily force the characters' actions and choices. Even though, say, Shakespeare's "will" for Hamlet transcends the world of the character, the melancholic Prince lives his life "freely."

Likewise, God, in His own sovereign and mysterious

---

[3] A prime example is the tautology "survival of the fittest." How do we know which species is the fittest? The one that survived. And why did it survive? Because it was the fittest, of course.

way, wills human persons to be as their First Cause while the secondary causes (AKA moms and dads) also act freely and according to the desires of their hearts. Beyond the human actors in the real-life drama called history stands the reality of God's providential plan. That God Himself causes human beings to be ought to cure our casual attitude toward preventing births. So when contraceptors say, "We don't want any more kids," our Bible-based reply ought to be, "And which of your kids don't you want?"

Heavenly Helpmate

> Now Adam knew Eve his wife, and she conceived and bore Cain, saying, "I have gotten a man *with the help of the Lord.*" . . . And Adam knew his wife again, and she bore a son and called his name Seth, for she said, "God has appointed for me another child instead of Abel, for Cain slew him." (Gen 4:1, 25)

> The Lord visited Sarah as he had said, and the Lord did to Sarah as he had promised. And Sarah conceived, and bore Abraham a son in his old age at the time of which God had spoken to him. (Gen 21:1–2)

> So Bo'az took Ruth and she became his wife; and he went in to her, and *the Lord gave her conception*, and she bore a son. (Ruth 4:13)

> Then Eli would bless Elka'nah and his wife, and say, "The Lord give you children by this woman for the loan which she lent to the Lord"; so then they would return to their home. *And the Lord visited Hannah,* and she conceived and bore three sons and two

daughters. And the boy Samuel grew in the presence of the Lord. (1 Sam 2:20–21)

After these days his wife Elizabeth conceived, and for five months she hid herself, saying, "Thus the *Lord has done to me* in the days when he looked on me, to take away my reproach among men." (Luke 1:24–25)

Miraculous Multiplier

The Bible consistently underscores God's "Author's rights" in the birth and multiplication of human beings. Here are some more examples:

- "The angel of the Lord also said to [Hagar], 'I will so greatly multiply your descendants that they cannot be numbered for multitude'" (Gen 16:10).
- "And I will make my covenant between me and you, and will multiply you exceedingly. . . . As for Ish'mael, I have heard you; behold, *I will bless him and make him fruitful and multiply him exceedingly*; he shall be the father of twelve princes, and I will make him a great nation" (Gen 17:2, 20).
- (God to Abraham): "I will indeed bless you, and *I will multiply your descendants* as the stars of heaven and as the sand which is on the seashore. And your descendants shall possess the gate of their enemies. . ." (Gen 22:17).
- (God to Isaac): "*I will multiply your descendants* as the stars of heaven, and will give to your descendants all these lands; and by your descendants all the nations of the earth shall bless themselves. . . . And

the Lord appeared to him the same night and said, 'I am the God of Abraham your father; fear not, for I am with you and will bless you and multiply your descendants for my servant Abraham's sake'" (Gen 26:4, 24).
- Genesis 28:3 (Isaac to his son Jacob): "*God Almighty bless you and make you fruitful and multiply you,* that you may become a company of peoples."
- Genesis 41:52: "The name of the second he called E'phraim, 'For *God has made me fruitful* in the land of my affliction.'"
- Genesis 48:3–4: "And Jacob said to Joseph, 'God Almighty appeared to me at Luz in the land of Canaan and blessed me, and said to me, 'Behold, *I will make you fruitful, and multiply you,* and I will make of you a company of peoples, and will give this land to your descendants after you for an everlasting possession.'"
- Exodus 32:13 (Moses to God): "Remember Abraham, Isaac, and Israel, thy servants, to whom thou didst swear by thine own self, and didst say to them, '*I will multiply your descendants as the stars of heaven,* and all this land that I have promised I will give to your descendants, and they shall inherit it for ever.'"
- Leviticus 26:9: "*I will have regard for you and make you fruitful and multiply* you, and will confirm my covenant with you."
- Deuteronomy 1:10–11 (Moses to the people): "*the Lord your God has multiplied you,* and behold, you are this day as the stars of heaven for multitude. May the Lord, the God of your fathers, make you a thousand times as many as you are, and bless you, as he has promised you!"
- Deuteronomy 28:63: "And as *the Lord took delight in*

doing you good and multiplying you, so the Lord will take delight in bringing ruin upon you and destroying you; and you shall be plucked off the land which you are entering to take possession of it."
- Deuteronomy 30:5: "and the Lord your God will bring you into the land which your fathers possessed, that you may possess it; and *he will make you more prosperous and numerous than your fathers.*"
- Joshua 24:3–4a (Joshua prophesying to the people): "Then I took your father Abraham from beyond the River and led him through all the land of Canaan, and made his offspring many. *I gave him Isaac; and to Isaac I gave Jacob and Esau.*"
- 1 Chronicles 27:23: "David did not number those below twenty years of age, for *the Lord had promised to make Israel as many as the stars of heaven.*"
- Psalm 105:24: "And *the Lord made his people very fruitful*, and made them stronger than their foes."
- Psalm 107:38: "*By his blessing they multiply greatly*; and he does not let their cattle decrease."
- Isaiah 26:15: "But *thou hast increased the nation, O Lord*; thou hast increased the nation; thou art glorified; thou hast enlarged all the borders of the land."
- Isaiah 51:2: "Look to Abraham your father and to Sarah who bore you; for when he was but one I called him, and *I blessed him and made him many.*"
- Jeremiah 30:19: "Out of them shall come songs of thanksgiving, and the voices of those who make merry. *I will multiply them, and they shall not be few*; I will make them honored, and they shall not be small."
- Jeremiah 33:22: "As the host of heaven cannot be numbered and the sands of the sea cannot be meas-

ured, so *I will multiply the descendants of David* my servant, and the Levitical priests who minister to me."

Barrenness and Blemishes

What about the flip side? How does the Bible treat sterility? To our modern ears, some of the biblical accounts sound harsh, even a little bizarre, especially in the Book of Leviticus. But blessings and curses are a recurrent Old Testament theme. The prophet Jeremiah identifies Yahweh's punishment with childlessness: "Therefore deliver up their children to famine; give them over to the power of the sword, let their wives become childless and widowed" (Jer 18:21).

The same theme is echoed later in Hosea:

> Like grapes in the wilderness, I found Israel; Like the first fruit on the fig tree, in its first season, I saw your fathers. But they came to Ba'al-pe'or, and consecrated themselves to Ba'al, and became detestable like the thing they loved. Ephraim's glory shall fly away like a bird—no birth, no pregnancy, no conception. . . . Give them, O Lord—what wilt thou give? Give them a miscarrying womb and dry breasts. (Hos 9:10–11, 14)

Leviticus 21:17 describes congenital sterility as a blemish in Israel's high priests (due to their special role in embodying God's holiness), and Deuteronomy 23:1 forbids men with crushed testicles or who are castrated from entering the assembly.

In preparing His chosen people for their entry into Canaan, the Lord promised the Israelites two blessings: protection from disease, and a complete absence of miscarriage and sterility (Exod 23:25–26), a promise renewed in Deuteronomy 7:13–14 immediately following the reception of the Ten Commandments. Traditional Judaism has always taught that a home without children is a home without blessing. Not surprisingly, there is no Old Testament word for bachelor. Sorrow is the universal emotion of childless Old Testament women.

Deuteronomy records an interesting prohibition: "When men fight with one another, and the wife of the one draws near to rescue her husband from the hand of him who is beating him, and puts out her hand and seizes him by the private parts, then you shall cut off her hand; your eye shall have no pity" (Deut 25:11–12). The editors of the *New Jerusalem Bible* tag this scene "Modesty in Brawls." Is that really all that is going on? As a moment's thought will verify, the wife had far less modest avenues available with which to intervene. What's at stake in protecting the integrity of the sex organs goes beyond merely fighting fairly. It's at least curious that there is no mention of punishment for grabbing or cutting off any other part of the enemy's body.

The Mosaic civil laws regulating sexual practice stem ultimately from a positive view of fertility. Leviticus 20 lists a number of sexual perversions that earned the death penalty: adultery and incest (Lev 10–12); sodomy (Lev 20:13); male-animal bestiality (Lev 20:15); and female-animal bestiality (Lev 20:16). The first ten verses of Leviticus 20 prescribe death for anyone "who gives any of his children to Molech" (v. 2)—the ancient equivalent of being offered up to a Planned Parenthood clinic.

This is not to imply that the Mosaic punishments, along with dietary restrictions, are still in force. They are not. The Old Law, with its ritual purities and strict sanctions for the sake of community order, was fulfilled by the coming of Christ and is no longer binding in its minutiae.

Yet Christ did not throw out the baby of truth with the bath water of the old rituals, and neither does the Church. Contrasting Moses with Christ, the Letter to the Hebrews affirms the basic validity of the Mosaic moral logic: "For if the message declared by angels was valid and every transgression or disobedience received a just retribution, how shall we escape if we neglect such a great salvation?" (Heb 2:2–3). Jesus Himself said, "Think not that I have come to abolish the law and the prophets; I have come not to abolish them but to fulfill them. For truly, I say to you, till heaven and earth pass away, not an iota, not a dot, will pass from the law until all is accomplished" (Matt 5:17–18).

The Unshod and the Dead

For those looking for scriptural evidence for the Catholic teaching against birth control, the granddaddy passage is the Onan incident in Genesis 38. Pius XI cites it in *Casti Connubii* (1930), which, in turn, is referenced in *Humanae Vitae* (1968). For Protestant "protesters" of birth control, the Onan episode is proof positive of God's abhorrence of the practice.

The context of the story can be pictured as three concentric circles with the Onan incident at the center. Moving outward, the next circle is the ancient Hebrew custom called the law of the Levirate, which obligated a brother to marry his dead brother's widow to carry on the family line of the deceased. (More on that shortly.) The third contextual circle is the way the passage has been understood by the Catholic Church and, as we've seen, by all Protestants for five hundred years before 1930. The following analysis draws on the work of Brian Harrison, OS, STD,[4] and John Kippley.[5] But before we look at the context, here is the text:

> It happened at that time that Judah went down from his brothers, and turned in to a certain Adul′lamite, whose name was Hirah. There Judah saw the daughter of a certain Canaanite whose name was Shua; he married her and went in to her, and she conceived and bore a son, and he called his name Er. Again she conceived and bore a son, and she called his name Onan. Yet again she bore a son, and she called his name Shelah. She was in Chezib when she bore him. And Judah took a wife for Er his first-born, and her name was Tamar. But Er, Judah's first-born, was wicked in the sight of the Lord; and the Lord slew him. Then Judah said to Onan, "Go in to your brother's wife, and perform the duty of a brother-in-law to her, and raise up offspring for your brother." But Onan knew that the offspring would not be his; so when he went in to his brother's wife he *spilled the semen on the ground*, lest he should give offspring to his brother. And *what he did* was *displeasing* in the sight of the Lord, and he slew him also." (Gen 38:1–10)

The Onan story interrupts a broader narrative, the story of Joseph, one of the sons of Jacob by Rachel. Chapter 37 ends with Jacob's tears over what he believes, falsely, is Joseph's death. Chapter 39 picks up the story with Joseph

---

[4] Fr. Brian W. Harrison, "The Sin of Onan Revisited," *Living Tradition* (67), November, 1996.
[5] John F. Kippley, "The Sin of Onan: Is It Relevant to Contraception?" *Homiletic and Pastoral Review,* 107 (2007): 16–22.

enjoying the Lord's special protection in Egypt under Potiphar. The Onan story is wedged between. One might say that Joseph's fratricidal brothers may have wished, in a manner of speaking, that their father Jacob had practiced Onanism with Rachel.

To review, Onan was the son of Judah and his Canaanite wife Shua, and the nephew of Joseph. He also had an elder brother, Er, and a junior brother, Shelah, the latter of whom had been recently slain by God for an undisclosed sin (many rabbinical commentators say it was the same as Onan's). Judah requests that Onan "go into" the childless Tamar (Er's widow) according to the standard custom of the Levirate law.[6] Resentful that the child would not be his, whenever they had relations, he deceptively ejaculated outside her body ("he spilled the semen upon the ground"). This rendering does not capture the force of the Hebrew verb *shichet*, which means not to spill or waste, but to act perversely.

Further, what earned Onan the punishment of death wasn't his intentions, feelings, or motives. It was his *action*, as verse 10 makes clear: "And what he did [*asher asah* in Hebrew] was displeasing in the sight of the Lord, and he slew him also." That's the Revised Standard Version. "Displeasing" is translated elsewhere as "offensive" (New Jerusalem Bible), "wicked" (New International Version, King James, Douay-Rheims), "evil" (American Standard Version), and *detestabilem* (Latin Vulgate).

The Onan passage, incidentally, is the basis for the Orthodox Jewish prohibition of condoms and any "spilling of the seed." There is a disarmingly obvious point to the passage: Onan was struck dead because he withdrew from an act of

---

[6] The Levirate tradition is also present in the Book of Ruth, and is also clearly on the minds of the Sadducees who question Jesus about who is married to whom in the Resurrection (Matt 22:23–32).

intercourse and ejaculated outside Tamar's body. The most common attempt at getting around this commonsensical conclusion is the claim that Onan was punished for evading his brotherly duty vis-à-vis the Levirate Law, or for failing to give Tamar what she was owed.

But the "Levirate breach only" interpretation does not work. First of all, God is never presented in Scripture as a capricious deity who doles out capital punishment for minor infractions or human foibles.

Second, as mentioned, the key verse (v. 10) refers specifically to what Onan *did,* to his act of withdrawal. And note that verse nine indicates that his relations with Tamar were an ongoing affair and not a one-night stand. The Revised Standard Version cited above uses the word "when" ("*when he went in to his brother's wife*") but the sense of the original Hebrew is *whenever,* which is the way it appears in the New American Bible, and others as well. Onan was repeatedly using his brother's widow for his own pleasure.[7]

Third, and most important, there was indeed a punishment for violating the Law of the Levirate, and you can find it in Deuteronomy 25 (see below). If a brother declined to have relations with his late brother's widow, she could subject him to a ritual of humiliation in which she would spit in his face, take off his sandals, and call him "House of the Unshod of Israel." While the Levirate custom was pro-life and had many practical benefits, Onan's sin was not merely to violate it (which he did!). After all, both Onan's father and his other

---

[7] Protestant scholar S. R. Driver pointed out that the verse should be understood as a frequentative use of the perfect and translated "whenever he went in" instead of "when he went in." See S. R. Driver, *The Book of Genesis* (New York: Edwin S. Gorham, 1905), 328; Ronald J. Williams, *Hebrew Syntax: An Outline*, 2nd ed. (Toronto: University of Toronto Press, 1976), 85; E. Kautzsch, ed., *Gesenius' Hebrew Grammar*, rev. ed., A. E. Cowley (Oxford: Clarendon Press, 1910), 336.

brother Shelah were also guilty of violating the Levirate law, but their chosen means of evasion were not contraceptive.

No, the key difference is that Onan went through the motions of fulfilling his family duty and yet withheld the very element that would have made him faithful to it. Here is the text:

> If brothers dwell together, and one of them dies and has no son, the wife of the dead shall not be married outside the family to a stranger; her husband's brother shall go in to her, and take her as his wife, and perform the duty of a husband's brother to her. And the first son whom she bears shall succeed to the name of his brother who is dead, that his name may not be blotted out of Israel. And if the man does not wish to take his brother's wife, then his brother's wife shall go up to the gate to the elders, and say, "My husband's brother refuses to perpetuate his brother's name in Israel; he will not perform the duty of a husband's brother to me." Then the elders of his city shall call him, and speak to him: and if he persists, saying, "I do not wish to take her," then his brother's wife shall go up to him in the presence of the elders, and pull his sandal off his foot, and spit in his face; and she shall answer and say, "So shall it be done to the man who does not build up his brother's house." And the name of his house shall be called in Israel, the house of him that had his sandal pulled off. (Deut 25:5–10)

Embarrassing and unpleasant, but hardly the death penalty. Notice the blunt description in Genesis 38, verse nine, "he spilled the semen on the ground." The only other biblical reference to the "spilling of seed" is in Ezekiel's prophetic allegory of the infidelities, rendered by the *New International Version* as: "There she lusted after her lovers, whose genitals were like those of donkeys and whose emission was like that of horses" (Ezek 23:20). (Chances are pretty good that this passage has never been preached on, even by the most daring preachers!)

Perversion vs. Purity

Whenever sexual perversion is treated in the Word of God, the language tends to be graphic, sordid. We read of "uncovering nakedness" (the Hebrew word is *galah*, a blunt term meaning to denude or forcefully strip). Then there is "nakedness" in a shameful sense (e.g., Gen 9:21–23; Isa 47:3; Ezek 16:37).[8]

A whole study could be done on the Bible's language for sexual sin. But for our purposes, it is enough to note that the nth degree of this verbal bluntness is reached with the use of the Hebrew verb *shagal*, which is found in Deuteronomy 28:30, Isaiah 13:16, Jeremiah 3:3, Zechariah 14:2, and nowhere else in Scripture. *Shagal* is the Hebrew equivalent of the vulgar English term for intercourse (the one that begins with an f). As a result, when *shagal* was read aloud, the Jews substituted it with *shakab*, meaning violate.[9] *Shakab* also

---

[8] For a fuller overview of the Bible's treatment of sexual sin, see Manuel Miguens, OFM, *Biblical Reflections on "Human Sexuality"* in *Human Sexuality in Our Time: What the Church Teaches*, ed. George A. Kelly (Jamaica Plain, MA: Daughters of Saint Paul, 1979) 102–118.

[9] Blue Letter Bible, "Dictionary and Word Search for *shagal* (Strong's 7693)," *Blue Letter Bible*, 1996–2010, http://www.blueletterbible.org/lang/lexicon/lexicon.cfm?Strongs=H7693&t=KJV (accessed September 26, 2009). A note of thanks to Fr. Mitch Pacwa, SJ, for this insight.

appears in Genesis 19:34–35 to describe inter-generational incest.

By contrast, whenever Scripture speaks of wholesome sexual activity, it invariably uses gentle, poetic terms that respect the private nature and true dignity of sex as God intended it. There is the beautiful eroticism of the Song of Songs, of Adam "knowing" Eve to produce their son Cain (Gen 4:1), and the Blessed Mother's reply to the angel, "How can this be, since I have no husband?" (Luke 1:34).

One of the last books of the Old Testament, the Book of the Prophet Malachi, harkens back to the first, Genesis. Malachi reminds his hearers that marriage is not merely a social contract but a covenant, a sacramental exchange of persons with children as its fruit:

> the Lord was witness to the covenant between you and the wife of your youth, to whom you have been faithless, though she is your companion and your wife by covenant. Has not the one God made and sustained for us the spirit of life? And what does he desire? Godly offspring. (Mal 2:14–15)

The final passage of Malachi's last chapter points forward to the arrival of John the Baptist, the "hinge" between the two Covenants, and to the coming of the New Moses, Jesus Christ. The restoration of families is expressed—not unlike the Book of Leviticus—in language that manages to be at once tough and tender:

> Remember the law of my servant Moses, the statutes and ordinances that I commanded him at Horeb for all Israel. Behold, I will send you Eli'jah the prophet before the great and terrible day of the Lord comes.

And he will turn the hearts of fathers to their children and the hearts of children to their fathers, lest I come and smite the land with a curse. (Mal 4:4–6)

Everything New Is Old Again

The New Testament carries forward the implicitly anti-contraceptive outlook of the Old Testament. To borrow from the popular adage, Jesus Christ had a preferential option for children. He pointed to children as models of Christian maturity and stressed the hospitality we must bear toward them. "Whoever receives one such child in my name receives me. . . . See that you do not despise one of these little ones; for I tell you that in heaven their angels always behold the face of my Father who is in heaven" (Matt 18:5, 10; see also 18:1–10, 19:13–15; Mark 10:13–16). The theme of childlikeness is key to Christian identity and is a constant in the writings of the saints and doctors of the Church.

One of Jesus' most pointed rebukes to His disciples concerned welcoming infants. "Now they were bringing even infants to him that he might touch them; and when the disciples saw it, they rebuked them. But Jesus called them to him, saying, "Let the children come to me, and do not hinder them; for to such belongs the kingdom of God" (Luke 18:16).

In biblical studies, the term *sensus plenior* (Latin for "fuller sense") refers to the deeper meaning God intended by a passage, which is rooted in—but not limited to—what the human author intended. Might not the Lord's vehement response to children being prevented from coming to Him have a more-than-literal meaning? Could He have been referring to children who would "come to Him" through the unsterilized sex acts of His followers through time until He returns?

Since He is the Word through whom all things are made (including babies; see John 1:1–3), it seems logical to see a parallel between the disciples' *hindering* of the infants and the *hindering* that is the essence of contraception.

The writings of St. Paul develop and deepen what is implicit in the Gospel. On the subject of Christian marriage in Ephesians 5:21–33, he teaches that wives ought to be submissive to their husbands "as to the Lord," while also emphasizing that the husband is to love his wife "as Christ loved the church," which is to say, by giving his entire self—body and soul—to her. The passage is, in fact, recommending the opposite of female slavery and male tyranny. The interpretive key here is the phrase "as to the Lord." The wife's submission (which means "ordered under") to the love and sacrificial mission of her husband in no way implies her inferiority. They are utterly equal and are equally called to "give way" to one another out of love for Christ. Christ Himself was submissive to His Father while remaining equal to Him.

The union of husband and wife is therefore a mirror of Christ's union with His Bride. At a minimum, this means that the bodily surrender in sexual intercourse must not be tainted by a clinging to self. To simultaneously say with one's body, "I give you my all," and, "I hold back my all," is the height of sexual schizophrenia. As we will see in Chapter Five, in His consummation of His marriage vows upon the cross—the ultimate exemplar of love's willingness to self-donate—Christ held nothing back.

Final Converging Clues

St. Paul's writings often address certain errors floating around in the community. In 1 Timothy 2:15, he probably had in mind those false teachers who forbade marriage (see

4:3). The apostle's conviction that "woman will be saved through bearing children" is a clear affirmation of motherhood as integral to married life, and a strong clue as to how the early Church valued fertility. While not an explicit "thou shalt not contracept," it is another sign that the New Testament viewed marriage as bound up with motherhood. If some birth control is morally okay, then what could be wrong with marriage entirely characterized by it to the point of deliberate childlessness? This would seem to contradict Paul's whole point.

In the original Greek, the New Testament also contains several references to *pharmakeia*, which is translated variously as sorcery, medicine, or drugs associated with magic (Gal 5:20; Rev 9:21, 18:23, 21:8, 22:15). The word carries overtones of the occult in connection with Babylonian practices, and many scholars identify *pharmakeia* with contraception, which was widely practiced by Israel's neighbors throughout history in Babylon, Egypt, Rome, and Greece. It is well-known that, in New Testament times, various potions were mixed to suppress or stop a pregnancy. Each mention of *pharmakeia* is set in the context of condemning sexual immorality and even murder (see Rev 9:21, 22:15). The early Church held a dim view of the first-century equivalent of the birth control pill.

The biblical injunctions against homosexual behavior are clearly set forth in both Testaments (see Gen 19:1–19; Lev 18:22–23, 20:13; Rom 1:24–32; 1 Cor 6:9). Sodomy in particular has something essentially in common with contraception; namely, sex without babies. From a strictly biological point of view, heterosexual couples who nullify their fertility through contraception (especially via sterilization) have dismantled the logical basis on which to criticize homosexual acts. The more honest and consistent Catholic dissenters have admitted that dissent from *Humanae Vitae* results in the logical acceptance (even if one subjectively finds them repellent) of many other perversions, including bestiality.[10]

Despite sincere protestations, those who accept contraception implicitly accept every other sexual coupling that is shorn from conception.

There is a popular misconception that pits the allegedly wrathful God of the Old Testament against the merciful God of the New. The *Cliff's Notes* version of this Old Testament deity might be "God creates man and everything man does gets God angry." But this is a false dichotomy. The Father of Jesus is as concerned with justice as Yahweh was with mercy. The New Testament, in fact, records an instance where God metes out the death penalty, and its circumstances bring us full circle back to the Onan incident. It's found in Acts 5:1–11, the strange case of Ananias and Sapphira.

This seemingly devout couple misled Peter and the apostles about property holdings they were meant to share with the community. They slyly withheld a gift, as it were, and defrauded their solemn commitment as leaders of the Christian community just as Onan defrauded his solemn commitment (or covenant oath) to bring forth new life for his brother. Ananias and Sapphira—not unlike Onan—discovered the hard way how seriously God takes covenant oaths.

At face value, the text in Acts 5 has nothing to do with birth control, but the similarity lies in the fact of lying, of

---

[10] Michael Valente, *Sex: The Radical View of a Catholic Theologian* (New York: Bruce-MacMillan, 1970); Anthony Kosnik et al., *Human Sexuality: New Directions in American Catholic Thought* (New York: Paulist Press, 1977); Charles E. Curran, "Divorce in the Light of the Revised Moral Theology" (Notre Dame, IN: Fides, 1975), 77–78, cited in Ronald Lawler, OFM Cap, Joseph Boyle, Jr., and William E. May, *Catholic Sexual Ethics: A Summary, Explanation and Defense* (Huntington, IN: Our Sunday Visitor Publishing, 1998), 47.

giving the appearance of transparency and truthfulness while really engaging in a deception. Contraception likewise gives the appearance of openness toward the natural link with procreation while severing that same link.

In severing love from life, contraception does what God's Word never does.

Chapter Five

BIRTH CONTROL AND THE BLESSED TRINITY
The Implications of Divine Self-Gift

I have not even begun to think of unity when the Trinity bathes me in its splendor; I have not even begun to think of the Trinity when unity grasps me.
—St. Gregory Nazianzus

From God's revelation in Scripture, we now consider God as He is and unpack what the Blessed Trinity might have to do with birth control. At first glance, absolutely nothing. They barely belong in the same sentence, one being of heaven, the other of earth. The dogma of the Trinity, however, carries two implicit condemnations of contraception, both of which are related to imitating our Creator in the choices we make, particularly in the marital, sexual realm.

But before we explore them, a quick review of the grand old teaching will better show the correspondence between the life of the Trinity and the teaching of *Humanae Vitae*.

The Big Idea

Many people feel it's impossible, even pointless, to try to understand the Trinity. They feel it's either an unsolvable puzzle, like a square circle, or an abstraction up in the clouds somewhere. For others, it's an article of faith, and that's enough for them. "It's a mystery," they shrug, and turn back to the football game. But we were *made* to understand the Trinity. If we're going to spend eternity with God—and God says He is a Trinity—it's a good idea to learn as much as possible about what that means. If you were on a bus to Florence, wouldn't your visit be more enjoyable in proportion to how much you learned about art?

The mystery of the Trinity embraces every other mystery of faith: our creation, our identity in Christ, and our final destiny in heaven. It's the tantalizing secret God couldn't keep to Himself (Rom 16:25, 26), which, in the fullness of time, He sent His Son to reveal (Gal 4:4).

The early Church formulated the Trinitarian dogma, fittingly enough, over the course of three Ecumenical Councils, Nicea (325), Ephesus (431), and Chalcedon (451). The dogma may be summarized by saying that God is one divine nature (His *what*ness) which belongs to three divine Persons (His *who*ness). The Father is God, the Son is God, and the Holy Spirit is God; and none of the Persons is any of the other. One God, not three Gods. The First Person, the Father, we designate as Creator; the Second Person, the Son, we designate as Redeemer; and the Third Person, the Holy Spirit, we designate as Sanctifier. Or, the Father above; the Son beside; the Spirit within.[1]

---

[1] In his work *De Trinitate*, St. Augustine points out that the word "person" is derived from our imperfect knowledge of creatures, and is

While Christians, like Jews and Muslims, believe strictly in one God, this one God drops a hint early on about some kind of plurality within Himself. After creating the world and everything in it, God suddenly uses the first person plural when creating man. "Let us make man in our image, after our likeness" (Gen 1:26). This idea is repeated when sin enters the Garden. "Behold, the man has become like one of us, knowing good and evil" (Gen 3:22).[2]

Us? Our? With the coming of Christ and the New Testament witness to the divinity of the Holy Spirit, these murky hints of more-than-oneness were brought to full clarity.[3]

The Father loves the Son infinitely; the Son loves the Father infinitely in return. The infinite love of Father for Son, and Son for Father, "breathes" (spirates) a third infinite love, which is the Holy Spirit. According to the *Catechism*, "The Church confesses, following the New Testament, 'one God and Father *from whom* all things are, and one Lord Jesus Christ, *through whom* all things are, and one Holy Spirit *in whom* all things are'" (CCC 258, emphases mine).

That's the Trinity in a nutshell. It's the Big Idea of Chris-

---

used to describe the Trinity because it's the least inaccurate one to be used.

[2] A few more examples: Hebrews 1:8 identifies "the throne of God" in Psalm 45 as the Son. In Isaiah 6:8 we read, "I heard the voice of the Lord saying, 'Whom shall I send, and who will go for us?'" Isaiah 48:16 is spoken by God, who says, "And now the Lord God has sent me and his Spirit." Elihu tells Job, "The Spirit of God has made me; the breathe of the Almighty gives me life" (Job 33:3). In Acts 13:33, Paul tells his hearers that "the Son" mentioned in Psalm 2:7 refers to Jesus. Threeness is embedded everywhere in nature: three primary colors; three modes of time (past, present, and future); protons, neutrons, and electrons make up the atom. Examples could be multiplied.

[3] Full clarity does not mean perfect understanding. While the dogma crystallizes a revealed truth, it remains essentially and always a mystery of faith. Would a God who can be fully understood be worthy of worship?

tianity: not a picture to be imagined but a truth to be known, three Persons to be loved. (Religious works of art depicting the Trinity, despite noble motives and luminous beauty, haven't exactly done the inquiring mind a big favor. For only the Son is "representable" in visual form; the Father and the Holy Spirit are by definition formless and invisible. If all you learned about the Trinity was gleaned from stained glass depictions, you probably think the Father is an old guy with a long beard, the Son a young guy with a short beard, and the Spirit some kind of white bird in flight.[4])

On Earth As It Is in Heaven

So what does any of this have to do with contraception, let alone with condemning it? The answer has two facets, both of which bear upon our vocation to imitate, not just the triune God, but also the Word made flesh, Jesus Christ, especially in his supreme example of self-emptying. Call it an application of the natural law in Trinitarian attire.

This God wants us not just to imitate Him; He wants us! And He has a nature far above ours to share with us. "As he who called you is holy," writes St. Peter, "be holy yourselves in all your conduct; since it is written, 'You shall be holy, for I am holy'" (1 Pet 1:15, 16).[5] Jesus, the image of the invisi-

---

[4] Even the famous shamrock image for the Trinity is misleading because it separates the three Persons, as if the Father could look over and wave at, say, the Son or the Holy Spirit.

[5] Other key texts include: "Through these, he has bestowed on us the precious and very great promises, so that through them you may come to *share in the divine nature* . . ." (2 Pet 1:4); "For God did not call us to impurity, but to holiness" (1 Thess 4:7); "Strive for peace with everyone, and for that *holiness*, without which no one will see the Lord" (Heb 12:14); "He chose us . . . to be *holy* and without blemish before him" (Eph 1:4); "Since we have these promises, beloved, let us cleanse ourselves from every defilement of flesh and spirit, making

ble God (Col 1:15), introduced this idea by commanding us to do something that, on first blush, seems impossible: "Be perfect, as your heavenly Father is perfect" (Mt 5:48).

Of our own feeble resources, obviously, we can do no such thing. Jesus asks us to do our best, but more importantly, as the Offertory at Mass hints, to let Him do His best *in us*: "By the mystery of this water and wine may we come to share in the divinity of Christ, who humbled himself to share in our humanity."

Biological fecundity is the physical echo of God's superabundant spiritual fecundity within the Godhead. His life is an eternal relation of three perfect self-donations, which are best understood not by what each keeps, but by what each *gives*: fatherhood, sonship, and the means to become holy. "God does as God is," as Forrest Gump might have reversed it.

In the Book of Genesis, sexual intercourse follows immediately upon creation.[6] The man (*ish*) and the woman (*ishshah*) become one flesh ("Adam knew Eve" Gen 4:1). With the birth of Cain, they are constituted as three. From one comes two; these two become one; and then the unity of the couple produces the "third" person of the child. Hence, the new husband-wife-child community is a dim, but real, reflection of God as Trinity, the transcendent "first family."

Like Father, Like Sons and Daughters

As we saw in Chapter Four, the Bible's first command is to "be fruitful and multiply" (note: not "be barren and divide").

---

holiness perfect in the fear of God" (2 Cor 7:1, *The New American Bible*, emphases mine).

[6] Only after the creation of man does God describe His work as "very good," i.e., exceedingly like Him.

This mandate comes in the very next verse after man is created (Gen 1:28). Made in God's image, man is called to respect his innate orientation toward new life—most particularly in the domain in which he's most profoundly the image of God in the co-creation of new life.

Why? Because all that touches upon life is sacred, because life has its source in God; an instinctive respect surrounds it.[7] When husband and wife become one flesh, a holy act takes place, which God may bless with the creation of a "someone" who will live forever in the kingdom of God. Endless permutations of future progeny are unleashed by a sexual act so blessed. We take hold of a whole series of events yet to be when we enter into that natural holy of holies that is sacramental genital union. We get a sideways glimpse at this mystery in Frank Capra's movie classic, *It's a Wonderful Life*, in which everyman hero George Bailey gets to see his world had he not existed.

When couples treat this mystery as a danger they cannot enter without "protection," then they unwittingly don a kind of invisible spiritual condom against the fecundity of the Holy Spirit.[8] This is not hyperbole. It's a consequence of the sin of contraception, which, objectively, always involves grave matter. To willingly refuse the gift of children while engaging in the act God designed for that purpose is

---

[7] The idea of procreation is closely tied with creation itself in many ancient languages, including Hebrew, the Old Testament's mother tongue. The verb *banah* (to make or construct, per Gen 2:22) is connected etymologically with *ben* (son); the verb *qanah* can mean both "create" (Gen 14:19) or "procreate" (Gen 4:1). *Bara* (technically, "to create") is related to the Aramaic *bar* (son). See P. van Imschoot, *Theologie de l'Ancien Testament*, vol. 2, 204–208, cited in Pierre Grelot, *Man and Wife in Scripture* (New York: Herder and Herder, 1964), 18.

[8] This also applies to the Pill, by which the woman chemically stops her generative faculty.

bound up in some way with refusing the gift of divine filiation from above. Fearing conception, yet unwilling to bridle their sexual urge for a short time, their union is no longer *life*-making.

It's a mutual grasping at an orgasm, the main liturgical action of worship of the false god mentioned in Chapter One.

All analogies limp, but hopefully this one is not a paraplegic: Imagine a hiker covered in smelly grime from hiking in the heat of the day. He has grown used to, and now defends his filthiness and ignores the pleading of his family to clean himself up. Suppose he's told about a sparkling waterfall that is fed by a beautiful lake in the high forest above.

The mud and the grime stand for personal sin; the day's heat, original sin; his defense of filthiness, pride; his pleading family, the Church. The lake is the Father; the waterfall is the Son "descending" to share his divine nature; and the invisible tug of gravity that draws the torrent down from the lake is the Holy Spirit, who brings us into relationship with the Father and the Son. And contraception? It would be unfurling a huge umbrella before stepping into the falling water—refusing to be cleansed yet grabbing at the sensation of refreshment, and treating the (objective) cleansing quality of the water as mere mist to luxuriate in.

Seen against the dynamism of life within the Trinity, as long as a marriage is characterized by birth control, it is tainted with a death wish—not wishing the death of an existent child, of course, but the metaphysical wish of imagining the prospect of a child and then taking positive steps to kill off his or her coming to be. The "me first" mentality is lethal to the family. If children are the fruit of marriage, then killing off the fruit at its source harms in a certain way the trunk and the root (i.e., the marital friendship and the vow that makes it a sacrament). No wonder so many "protected" marriages die anyway, and from a direction they never saw coming.

Again, notice the very word contraception. Its *raison d'être* is to be in opposition, always against something or someone. It targets the imagined-as-being-conceived child whose debut they have considered as possible, and then sabotaged.

We took the long way, but we have arrived at the first implicit indictment of contraception: it contradicts God's Trinitarian model of self-donation by turning the direction of love as envisioned by *Humanae Vitae* back upon the self, instead of toward the lover/beloved.

Here Comes the Bridegroom

The second link between the Trinity and the message of *Humanae Vitae* expresses the same thing more vividly. It's the radical example of the Son, our Lord Jesus Christ, considered especially as the Bridegroom in His sacred passion.

The words of the Nicene Creed summarize what He did "for us men and for our salvation;" they also provide concrete ideals for husbands to meditate upon. The Creed skips past the details of Our Lord's life, and announces that "He was born of the Virgin Mary," and then "suffered under Pontius Pilate, was crucified, died, and was buried."

The mind of St. Paul seems to have been on fire with the terrible beauty of this self-emptying (*kenosis*) when he described a kind of primitive inkling of the Trinity:

> [He], though he was *in the form of God*, did not count *equality with God* a thing to be grasped, but emptied himself, taking the form of a servant, being born in the likeness of men. And being found in human form

he *humbled himself* and *became obedient* unto death, even death on a cross. (Phil 2:6–8)

Kimberly Hahn has a lovely description of this act of nuptial union and communion:

> Love leads to life; life leads to sacrifice. Jesus does in the flesh what He has always done in his divinity: He loves with complete self-donation. Of course the difficulty with loving with complete self-donation is that it requires the ultimate sacrifice of life in death. When Jesus took on human flesh in the Incarnation, His self-offering involved His life, death, and resurrection as the supreme gift of His love for us. It is this self-offering that He took into the Holy of Holies in heaven when He ascended to the Father (see Heb 9:11–14).[9]

This sacrifice was not done as a judge for a plaintiff, or a warrior for a king, but as a bridegroom for his bride. According to the apostle Paul, the marital embrace is the pre-eminent earthly symbol to describe the indescribable union between Christ and His Church (Eph 5:31–33). Paul builds upon the bridal imagery foreshadowed in the Old Testament where God's love for Israel is likened to a husband's love for his bride (see Isa 61:10–11; Hos 2:16–20; Song of Solomon, etc.). It also appears later in St. John's apocalyptic vision: "And I saw the holy city, new Jerusalem, coming down out of heaven from God, prepared as a bride adorned for her husband.... Then came one of the seven angels who

---

[9] Kimberly Kirk Hahn, *Life-Giving Love: Embracing God's Design for Marriage* (Ann Arbor: Servant Publications, 2001), 93.

had the seven bowls full of the seven last plagues, and spoke to me, saying, 'Come, I will show you the Bride, the wife of the Lamb'" (Rev 21:2, 9).

Christopher West, accenting Pope John Paul's Theology of the Body, ties together the marital themes of both Testaments:

> Just as God organically inscribed the marital union of Adam and Eve in the mystery of creation, he organically inscribes the "marital" union of the new Adam and the new Eve (Christ and the Church) in the mystery of redemption. Spousal union, in fact, becomes the foundation upon which God constructs the entire mystery of our salvation in Christ.[10]

As the bridal, so the maternal. Christ constitutes the Church as Bride by Christ so she could become our Mother. This Mother then gives supernatural birth to new children by the "womb" of her baptismal font, so women share in this bridal maternity by being called to motherhood, whether spiritual or biological. St. Paul does not hesitate to say that "woman will be saved through bearing children" (1 Tim 2:15).

The "unbreakable connection" between the procreative and unitive meanings of the marital act taught by *Humanae Vitae* is the logical outgrowth of Jesus' teaching of the indissolubility of marriage in Matthew 19:5–6, which harkened back to the way it was "in the beginning." For the invisible love of husband for wife, and wife for husband, is so charged with promise that the two *do* become one in a breathtakingly literal way—in the form of a diaper-clad nap

---

[10] Christopher West, *Theology of the Body for Beginners* (West Chester, PA: Ascension Press, 2004), 87.

enthusiast! From this angle, every child is a kind of Incarnation in miniature.[11]

Taking a provocative step further, St. Augustine referred to the cross as the marriage bed of Christ. "Like a bridegroom Christ went forth from his chamber, he went out with a presage of his nuptials into the field of the world," wrote the saint of Hippo. "He came to the marriage bed of the cross, and there, in mounting it, he consummated his marriage. And where he perceived the sighs of the creature, he lovingly gave himself up in place of his bride, and he joined himself to the woman forever."[12]

Augustine's comparison is worth lingering on. On a symbolic level, does it not intimate something of the outlook we ought to have toward the life-bedecked consequences of each act of intercourse? More, if the cross stands for Christ's mystical marriage bed, and consummation refers to His saving death, what kind of grotesque sacrilege would contraception signify? It would be Jesus ensuring in secret that His death on the cross was faked, that it did not really save us, in other words, the Bridegroom defrauding His Bride in a convincing, and satanic, lie.

This Is My Body, Which Is Kept from You?

Of course, any reference to the intention of the Bridegroom will also have a eucharistic meaning. And here, too, birth control is tacitly rejected. Two key prophecies about Jesus—the suffering servant (Isa 53) and the gentle lamb (Jer

---

[11] From the perspective of generation within the Trinity, the title of child is appropriated to the Incarnate Word, the Son. But from the perspective of procession, the child role also is appropriated to the Holy Spirit, who "proceeds from the Father and the Son."

[12] St. Augustine of Hippo, *Sermo Suppositus*, 120, 8.

11:19)—are both realized in the Eucharist, the fulfillment of the ancient Jewish tradition of sacrificing an unblemished lamb for the Passover Seder meal (Exod 12).

In the Eucharist, the bread and wine are changed into the Body and Blood, soul and divinity of Jesus Christ. When we consume the Lamb of God "who takes away the sins of the world" (John 1:29), we enter into the closest possible encounter with Him this side of heaven. Jesus' high priestly prayer for unity in John 14 comes literally true as He abides in us that we might abide in Him. The ecstatic sexual union of marriage is a foretaste, however gauzy and pale, of the eternal love-union God "has prepared for those who love Him" (1 Cor 2:9).

It is easy to forget that our Lord could have saved us at the Last Supper by speaking a word or snapping a finger. Yet He willed that the Supper of Holy Thursday should be joined with the Sacrifice of Good Friday, and plunged Himself into a horrific experience of abandonment and torture, unto a messy death no crime writer ever dreamed of. Why? To demonstrate "to the end" (CCC 1337) His total communion with us, even amidst unimaginable suffering and its terminus in death. Atheists and other scoffers can no longer say, "God doesn't understand."

Peter Kreeft explains the relationship between repast and redemption against this Trinitarian background:

> It is a banquet because it is a sacrifice, just as any earthly food can be eaten only because it is first killed and "offered" to eat. Whether animal or vegetable, its natural life is ended, given up to nourish the life of the one who eats it. "My life for yours"—this is the law of nature and of grace. It is even the life of glory. Self-donation, the ecstatic coming out of the self and

giving of the self in love, is the essence of our eternal life in heaven, because that is our sharing in the very life of the Trinity.[13]

In the Eucharist, we receive the Body of God into our bodies. The Eucharistic Bridegroom impregnates us, as it were, with His divine life so that we can become other Christs for the world. "You are what you eat."

But what if a man in the communion line inserted a latex sheath into his mouth (like the ones used by the dentist when filling a tooth) before going up to receive Holy Communion so that the Host wouldn't be truly received? This is analogous of the condom writ Eucharistic. Or what if a woman swallowed something beforehand that would cause vomiting and ensure that the Host would be purged before truly entering her body? This parallels the Pill. Don't these anti-eucharistic actions bring to mind the word *blasphemy*?

I Love You, But . . .

Birth control causes, and is caused by, a schizoid attitude toward life. It loves journeys, the wild seas, and jokes—and hates destinations, safe harbors, and conclusions.[14] By spurning the example of our divine Bridegroom, it *puts asunder* the twofold meanings of love and life that God has joined together in the marital act. It throws each spouse back upon

---

[13] Peter Kreeft, PhD, *Catholic Christianity: A Complete Catechism of Catholic Beliefs Based on the Catechism of the Catholic Church* (San Francisco: Ignatius Press, 2001), 330.

[14] The "condom nation" culture, with its fruitless search for "more" (hotter sex, cheaper Viagra, better silicone, etc.), has reaped a harvest of impotence, sub-replacement population levels, and a high divorce rate, proving once and for all that "free love" not only costs—it collects.

self, instead of outward in generosity. The best it can say for itself—the banner it marches under—is, "I love you, but . . ."

One woman who knew the Trinity on a "first Names" basis was Blessed Mother Teresa of Calcutta. At the 1994 National Prayer Breakfast in Washington, DC, she described how birth control epitomizes the Pyrrhic victory of Me over We. "In destroying the power of giving life through contraception," she told the rapt audience of world leaders, "a husband and wife are doing something to self. This turns attention to self, and so it destroys the gift of love in him or her."

Chapter Six

CONTRACEPTION AND THE NATURAL LAW

What the law requires is written on their hearts.
—Romans 2:15

From the Trinitarian heights we return to *terra firma* to examine a very concrete idea that nourishes the mind of the Church in many moral disputes.

The arguments traditionally employed against contraception (while strongly attested to by Scripture) are not exclusively dependent upon Revelation, and in fact have nothing directly to do with a particular religion. This is partly why, compared with other papal encyclicals, *Humanae Vitae* cites relatively few Bible verses. The Church's opposition to contraception is based mainly on what is called the natural law. What is the "natural law"?

The Impossible-Not-to-Be-Known Law

Natural law is sometimes mistaken for the laws of nature, such as the growth of plants, the birth of stars, or the migration of moose. It really means the rule of conduct prescribed to us by the Creator in and through the way He made us. It sounds a bit abstract at first, but it's simple and practical. Natural law refers to that which rational beings must do in order to perfect their natures.

Take an example from the inanimate world. To properly operate a toaster according to its nature, you must insert sliced bread, not a cardboard fake. The cardboard may look like toast, and inserting it may feel so right, but the result will be decidedly untasty. Or say you're baking a cake and, owing to your fondness for the word "strychnine," you add a pinch into the cake mix. All positive feelings for the poison are cancelled by its actual presence in one's food.

As the nature of toasters and strychnine must be respected in the culinary sphere, so the nature of human actions—particularly, for our purposes, sexual intercourse—must be respected in the moral sphere if things are to go well for us.

The pioneering expositor of natural law analysis is St. Thomas Aquinas (+1274). According to Aquinas, the natural law is "nothing else than the rational creature's participation in the eternal law" (*Summa* I-II, Q. 94). This eternal law is God's wisdom, and He lovingly willed that we should somehow participate in it through conscience in the way we live our lives; its supreme rule is that what is genuinely fulfilling for human beings must be respected (see *Summa* I-II, Q. 94, art. 2.).

Extending the teaching of his ancient mentor, Aristotle, St. Thomas starts from the premise that goodness is what our human nature naturally seeks; so, the first principle of moral action must have the Good as its main idea—not what feels good, looks good, or smells good, but what is really good for us. (Tequila may keep my back pain at bay for a while, but I really need a chiropractor.)

Natural law refers to "the right thing to do," the moral rule of right and wrong we cannot not know. Actions that respect the basic goods to which our nature inclines us, and thus cooperate with God's wise plan for creation, are right and morally good; those that in one way or another denigrate a basic good, and thus thwart God's directives, are wrong and morally bad.

Dualism and Its Discontents

Two main impediments prevent people from clearly seeing the workings of the natural law in human affairs; and much of society has adopted both, almost by osmosis. The first is dualism.[1] The other is relativism.

According to dualism, the "true self" is identified solely with the mind or with consciousness. The body is seen as an extrinsic add-on, like a sock to a foot. It's valid to speak of *my* body, as opposed to yours, but the dualist sees the body more as inert property, something radically separated from the "real" inner person.

An old TV ad warned, "It's not nice to fool Mother Nature." A dualist culture wants every day to be April Fool's Day on Mother. For we no longer look upon our bodies and see evidence of a Designer—only a blank slate on which to write ourselves, edit ourselves, or, if need be, delete ourselves by euthanasia. We indelibly (and painfully) paint ourselves with tattoos. We stick rings into our nostrils and navels, and create specialized cosmetic surgeries to fix imperfections

---

[1] Dualism disposes us to see our body parts as machine-like cogs that can be adjusted, snipped, or removed in a morally neutral way for any motive of the "real self" who "owns" them. According to dualism, a person in an irreversible coma ("the grandpa we remember") is deemed no longer to be meaningfully present in the body, and is therefore marked for termination.

that were not so long ago thought to be assets. We nip and tuck because we can. (As a description of the influence of dualism, this is a short list.²)

The vision of Scripture is far from such a mechanized, imperialistic view of our bodies. "Do you not know that your body is a temple of the Holy Spirit within you . . . you are not your own; you were bought with a price" (1 Cor 6:19–20). Classical philosophy has always held that the body is an integral aspect of the person. On this view, in the words of John Paul II, "The body, in fact, and it alone is capable of making visible what is invisible, the spiritual and divine. It was created to transfer in the visible reality of the world, the invisible mystery hidden in God from time immemorial, and thus to be a sign of it" (General Weekly Audience, February 20, 1980).

Our society holds a schizoid view when it comes to protesting human tampering with nature. The environmental movement lectures aggressively that nature is inviolable when it comes to the earth's resources, to pollution, or global warming, and to the environment. Why doesn't the same principle apply to the environment of the human body? Who lops off a healthy finger or gouges out a functioning eyeball?

Another obstacle to seeing natural law as a workable theory of morality is relativism, the belief that right and wrong are either (a) matters of opinion; or (b) such bendy concepts that they can have no fixed meaning, such that what's right for you can be simultaneously wrong for me. While it's fashionable in college cafeterias, newsrooms, and discotheques to talk the "you have your truth, I have mine" talk, in the real world, no one really believes it. If you cut

---

² For a comprehensive treatment of dualism in theory and practice, see Patrick Lee and Robert P. George, *Body-Self Dualism in Contemporary Ethics and Politics* (Cambridge University Press: 2008).

the movie theater line in front of an ardent relativist, he responds, "Back of the line, buddy!" not, "Gosh, who's to know what's right or wrong?"

The Law of Nature and Nature's God

The natural law (sometimes called the moral law) applies not to animals or non-living things—only to mankind. "If a rock falls from a cliff and hits us on the head we do not punish it. We do not blame the pig for being greedy or reproach the leopard for its cruelty. It is in their nature to be that way. It is the law of their being. But when a human strikes us, or is greedy or cruel, we blame him and say he should act differently."[3] In other words, there's a certain standard of behavior human beings instinctively apprehend, even without having read a single line of high-fallutin' philosophizing about it. This is as true of atheists as of daily communicants.

And yet, as I emphasized in the introduction, any correct understanding of the natural law relative to something as culturally accepted as contraception is deeply affected by our fallen natures. In this area, to state the obvious, our erotomaniac culture stands in need of divine grace and the teaching of Christ. While natural law is objective and knowable by all, the kindly atheist is therefore less likely than the crotchety daily communicant to grasp the truth of *Humanae Vitae*.

The Second Vatican Council alludes to natural law in several key sections:[4]

---

[3] Daniel J. Sullivan, *Introduction to Philosophy: The Perennial Principles of the Classic Realist Tradition* (Rockford, IL: Tan Books, 1992), 140.
[4] I borrow here from the useful summary given by William E. May in *Introduction to Moral Theology* (Huntington, IN: Our Sunday Visitor, 1994), 43; 60–65.

- "It is in accordance with their dignity as persons—that is, beings endowed with reason and free will and therefore privileged to bear personal responsibility—that all men should be at once impelled by nature and also bound by a moral obligation to seek the truth."[5]
- "The highest norm of human life is the divine law—eternal, objective and universal—whereby God orders, directs and governs the entire universe and all the ways of the human community by a plan conceived in wisdom and love" (DH 3).
- "For the Church is, by the will of Christ, the teacher of the truth. It is her duty to give utterance to, and authoritatively to teach, that truth which is Christ Himself, and also to declare and confirm by her authority those principles of the moral order which have their origins in human nature itself" (DH 14; Paul VI builds on this passage in Section 4 of *Humanae Vitae*).
- Man discovers this law of God "in the depths of his conscience," and that this law summons man to "to love good and avoid evil" (GS 16).
- In reference to the Church's right and duty to proclaim the Gospel, "by imparting the knowledge of the divine and natural law" (GS 89).

Again, these sections express in technical language what we know from everyday life. No one delights in being lied to, or stolen from. If someone steals from our store, we don't sit down like Rodin's statue *The Thinker* and wonder

---

[5] Second Vatican Council, Declaration on Religious Freedom *Dignitatis Humanae* (December 7, 1965), § 2 (hereafter cited in text as *DH*).

if there is such a thing as an absolute morality. No, we call the cops.

The Appendix of *The Abolition of Man* by C.S. Lewis provides a review of moral maxims from wildly divergent human cultures. Lewis found that, with minor differences, what western philosophy calls the natural law is perceived universally. No known civilization has ever handed out trophies for cowardice, ribbons for corruption, or medals for mocking the blind.

The Truth Whisperer

The external natural law has an internal counterpart: man's built-in detection and decision apparatus known as conscience. The *Catechism* defines conscience as "a judgment of reason whereby the human person recognizes the moral quality of a concrete act that he is going to perform, is in the process of performing, or has already completed" (CCC 1778). Human conscience doesn't invent moral truth, nor does culture or socialization create it (although it does condition our sensitivity to it); conscience discovers it and urges us to act this way or that, according to the facts before us. Cardinal Newman called it the "aboriginal Vicar of Christ."

Conscience isn't a perfect means of perceiving moral truth, as we know, since fallen human nature is weak and limited. The voice of conscience doesn't imprint itself in our hearts and minds as unmistakably as it did "in the beginning," before sin entered the world. "Sin makes you stupid," as the saying goes. The whole concept of conscience has been hijacked to mean any sincere feeling about what one has done, is about to do, or wants to do.

St. Pope John Paul II warned against the temptation to be facile and self-serving when it comes to moral decision-making:

> As the Apostle Paul says, the conscience must be "confirmed by the Holy Spirit" (cf. Rom 9:1); it must be "clear" (2 Tim 1:3); it must not "practice cunning and tamper with God's word," but "openly state the truth" (cf. 2 Cor 4:2). On the other hand, the Apostle also warns Christians: "Do not be conformed to this world but be transformed by the renewal of your mind, that you may prove what is the will of God, what is good and acceptable and perfect" (Rom 12:2). Paul's admonition urges us to be watchful, warning us that in the judgments of our conscience the possibility of error is always present. Conscience *is not an infallible judge*; it can make mistakes.[6]

Paul told the Christians in Rome that this fallible grasp of natural law is the basis of accountability for the Gentiles, those who never received God's revealed law (Rom 1:32; 2:14–16). The natural law needed to be superseded and perfected by the supernatural, which was accomplished through the Incarnation. Ultimately, conscience can be a powerful ally in the spiritual battle. George Cardinal Pell of Sydney wrote, "The formation of a Christian conscience is thus a dignifying and liberating experience; it does not mean a resentful submission to God's law but a free choosing of that law as our life's ideal."[7]

---

[6] John Paul II, The Splendor of Truth *Veritatis Splendor* (August 6, 1993), § 62, emphasis in original.

[7] George Cardinal Pell, "The Inconvenient Conscience," *First Things*, (May 2005), 23.

CONTRACEPTION AND THE NATURAL LAW

From: Pope Paul
To: All

Pope Paul VI cites the teaching of four previous popes in affirming that the Church's interpretive competence is not restricted to divinely revealed spiritual matters, but includes the natural moral law as well:

> Let no one of the faithful deny that the Magisterium of the Church is competent to interpret the natural moral law. For it is indisputable—as our Predecessors have often declared—that when Jesus Christ imparted his divine authority to Peter and the other apostles and sent them to all nations to teach his Commandments, he established those very men as authentic guardians and interpreters of the whole moral law, that is, not only of the law of the Gospel, but also of natural law. For natural law (as well as revealed law) declares the will of God; thus faithful compliance with natural law is necessary for eternal salvation. (HV 4)

Here he is witnessing both to the constant self-understanding of the Catholic Church as the true guardian/interpreter of the natural law, and asserting that obedience to this law is necessary for eternal salvation. Another footnote in Section 4 invokes Christ's words, "Not everyone who says to me, 'Lord, Lord' shall enter the kingdom of heaven, but he who does the will of my Father who is in heaven" (Matt 7:21).

So the condemnation of birth control is not the oddball opinion of a past pope, nor a "ban" that some future pope could lift. Nor is it a custom relative to one's particular faith (e.g., Jews don't eat pork, Baptists don't dance, Catholics don't contracept). On the contrary, since Catholics aren't the only ones with a human nature, and aren't the only ones who propagate via sexual intercourse, this teaching is proposed equally to everyone as the truth. It's the opposite of sectarian; it's universal (*katholikos*).

In the eyes of the world, this is high scandal. Yet the Holy Father addressed *Humanae Vitae* to "all men of good will" and appealed to the very broad foundation of natural law as "illuminated and enriched by divine Revelation." As a good evangelist and teacher, he knew the natural correspondence between faith and reason, but also that God's Word boosts the candlepower of the natural law, so we may see it with brighter clarity and obey it with greater ease—joy, even.

Okay, enough setting the stage. How does the natural law apply to contraception?

How Natural Law Applies to Contraception

There is no single "official" way of understanding how contraception violates the natural law. Indeed, there are different, sometimes conflicting, theories held by Catholic scholars on this question. Assessing their differences would bring us far afield, but the mere fact of variation in approach is not an argument against the natural law, for all orthodox writers agree on the basic content.[8]

---

[8] For further treatments of the natural law from varying perspectives, see John Goyette, Mark S. Latkovic, Richard S. Myers, eds., *Saint Thomas Aquinas and the Natural Law Tradition: Contemporary Perspectives* (Washington: Catholic University of America Press: 2004); Janet E. Smith, *Humanae Vitae: A Generation Later* (Washington, DC: Catholic University Press of America, 1991), 69–128; J. Budziszewski, *Written on the Heart: The Case for Natural Law* (Downer's Grove, IN: InterVarsity Press, 1997); Germain Grisez, Joseph Boyle, and

For our purposes, it's enough to say that contraception violates the natural law because contraception acts against the natural end, or goal, of sexual intercourse, which is the coming to be of new human life. Sexual intercourse is, in Janet Smith's fine phrase, clearly ordained to "babies and bonding."[9] We tamper with this fundamental order of things at our peril.

Contraception is inherently anti-life because it treats a real good (the child-to-be) as undesirable enough to motivate a counter-action against the very possibility of its arrival in the womb. A well-functioning biological process is regarded as a threat to the pursuit of subjective pleasure at the expense of objective purpose.

One famous way of glimpsing the natural law in action is to consider the natural end, or purpose, of eating. Obviously, it is nutrition. The mouth, teeth, tongue, esophagus, stomach, and the rest of the digestive system comprise a set of organs and processes that are ordered to the purpose of maintaining nutritive health.

But food is also tasty (well, except for cauliflower), and it's pleasurable to enjoy a hearty meal with family and friends. Even if the food tasted awful, to stay alive you'd still eat it, i.e., you'd act in accord with reason in harmony with the natural law. We will revisit this analogy in Chapter Ten.

You can probably guess where this is going. Birth

John Finnis, "Practical Principles, Moral Truth and Ultimate Ends," in *American Journal of Jurisprudence* 32 (1987), 99–151; Russell Hittinger, *A Critique of the New Natural Law Theory* (Notre Dame, IN: University of Notre Dame Press, 1987); Saint Thomas Aquinas, Questions 91–94, I-II, in the *Summa Theologica*; C. S. Lewis, *The Abolition of Man* (New York: MacMillan, 1955).

[9] See Janet E. Smith, "Contraception: Why Not?" a compelling talk recorded and distributed by One More Soul (see Appendix to order a copy).

control (particularly the condom and coitus interruptus) corresponds to putting a spoon down one's throat to induce vomiting. The sensual pleasure of eating would thus be indulged in for its own sake, severed from its primary end, much like the Roman custom of feasting, stepping into the vomitorium to disgorge the food, and returning for more.

If human life is sacred and inviolable, then the means of transmitting human life is in some way sacred and inviolable. In a similar sense in which the eye was made for color, the ear for sound, and the mind for truth, sex was made for something: for the co-creation of a new someone, and the deepened unity of those (hopefully loving) co-creators otherwise known as mom and dad. The whole contraceptive enterprise denies this. Therefore, insofar as it meddles with a natural power that transcends both spouses, it is unnatural.[10]

Dr. Smith has summarized six different natural law arguments against contraception, which she dissects for validity and logical soundness.[11] Her Version D is the most similar to what we have said about the link between God's sacredness and the reverence we owe to His special involvement, so to speak, in the marital act:

- *Major premise*: It is wrong to impede the procreative power of actions that are ordained by their nature to assist God in performing His creative act that brings forth a new human life.

---

[10] A conspicuous exception to the idea that contraceptive behavior is always deliberately immoral ("meddling") would be a woman married to a tyrant or living in, say, a one-child-only dictatorship such as communist China. Smith points out that it's dubious at best to assume that such women are intentionally trying to avoid the burdens of motherhood.

[11] Smith, *Humanae Vitae*, 99, 102–104.

- *Minor premise*: Contraception impedes the procreative power of actions that are ordained by their nature to assist God in performing His creative act that brings forth a new human life.
- *Conclusion*: Therefore, contraception is wrong.

The key word is "impede." Contraception is sex—*plus* the introduction of an impediment. As we'll see later, abstinence during natural family planning is not an impediment in any sense since there is no sex act to impede.

Among other things, the above argument conveys something of the world's best-kept secret: the deep veneration the Catholic Church has toward sex.[12] The world has it exactly backwards. The world tends to look upon sex as merely currency for "hook-ups," as a proof of love, as something for sale—or, more commonly, something by which to sell something else, like cars or beer.

The Catholic Church turns this thinking right side up and proclaims that sexual intercourse—and all the erotic intimacies that cultivate it—deserves the most thoroughgoing protection and respect. "Casual sex" is an oxymoron. When a young man picks out a ring for his intended, he makes sure the ring and its setting matches the beauty of the diamond. He would never Krazy glue the diamond onto a plastic ring. And upon receiving her ring, the young fiancée would never toss it carelessly on a park bench or keep it near the edge of the toilet seat. We naturally, or ought to, treat as awesome things that fill us with awe.

Likewise, it is most fitting that sex be surrounded by the proper setting (the security of marriage), and within

---

[12] Veneration comes from the Latin verb *venerari*, meaning "to regard with great respect," and derives from the same root as Venus, the Roman goddess of love.

marriage, accorded the proper respect (freedom from the intrusion of contraception). Catholicism affirms that sex is not merely acceptable or tolerable ("close your eyes and think of England") but pure and holy—something that ought never be subject to the blessing-refusal inherent in contraception.

In every Christian wedding, we hear the words from Matthew's Gospel, "What God has joined let no man put asunder." But this is exactly what contraception does on the biological and interpersonal level. It puts asunder the two meanings of sex that God has joined, the unitive and the procreative.

The Heart of *Humanae Vitae*

The core principle of the encyclical—the hook upon which the whole garment hangs—is conveyed in one sentence: "The Church, nevertheless, in urging men to the observance of the precepts of the natural law, which it interprets by its constant doctrine, teaches that *each and every marital act must of necessity retain its intrinsic relationship to the procreation of human life*" (HV 11).

The above is from the official Vatican translation. (Although Latin is the official language of the Church, not all papal documents are originally written in Latin. Paul VI penned *Humanae Vitae* in Italian and French.) The Daughters of Saint Paul translation renders the italicized key phrase above as, "[The Church] teaches that each and every marriage act must remain open to the transmission of life." Dr. Smith's own version is: "[The Church] teaches that it is necessary that each conjugal act remain ordained in itself to the procreating of human life."

Like different camera angles used to shoot the same

scene, these renderings say the same basic thing, which is that the marital act—each and every one, not an aggregate "totality" of marital acts over the years—is ordained in itself to bring forth new human beings. Being the extraordinary site, so to speak, of God's interaction with His beloved co-creators, this act ought never be tainted by the ambushing of its potentialities.

Salvo across the Bow

Prior to *Humanae Vitae*, the major encyclical that addressed birth control was *Casti Connubii* ("On Christian Marriage"), issued by Pius XI[13] on December 31, 1930. It was the *de facto* Catholic response to the Anglican exit from the historic Christian position at the Lambeth Conference in August of that year; and, like *Humanae Vitae* twenty-eight years later, *Casti Connubii* invoked the natural law and the divine origins of the Church's role as Teacher, albeit in more muscular language:

> Since, therefore, the conjugal act is destined primarily by nature for the begetting of children, those who in exercising it deliberately frustrate its natural power and purpose sin against nature and commit a deed which is shameful and intrinsically vicious.
>
> Small wonder, therefore, if Holy Writ bears witness that the Divine Majesty regards with great-

---

[13] Born Achille Ratti, Pius XI was a kindred spirit of Pope John Paul II. Pius XI was a linguist, a scholar (obtaining three doctorates), and an avid mountain climber. Seeing the vast evangelistic potential in the nascent mass media, he started Vatican Radio in 1931 and became the first pope on the radio. In 1937, this proto-Wojtyla wrote the first papal condemnations of Nazism (*Mit Brennender Sorge*) and of Communism (*Divini Redemptoris*).

est detestation this horrible crime and at times has punished it with death. As St. Augustine notes, "Intercourse even with one's legitimate wife is unlawful and wicked where the conception of the offspring is prevented. Onan, the son of Judah, did this and the Lord killed him for it."

Since, therefore, openly departing from the uninterrupted Christian tradition some recently have judged it possible solemnly to declare another doctrine regarding this question, the Catholic Church, to whom God has entrusted the defense of the integrity and purity of morals, standing erect in the midst of the moral ruin which surrounds her, in order that she may preserve the chastity of the nuptial union from being defiled by this foul stain, raises her voice in token of her divine ambassadorship and through Our mouth proclaims anew: any use whatsoever of matrimony exercised in such a way that the act is deliberately frustrated in its natural power to generate life is an offense against the law of God and of nature, and those who indulge in such are branded with the guilt of a grave sin. (CC 54–6)

Notice the vehement language. "Shameful," "intrinsically vicious" (i.e., strongly attached to vice), "horrible crime," "moral ruin," "foul stain," "offense against the law of God," "branded with the guilt of a grave sin."[14] Could two papal writing styles be more different? Paul VI was criticized

---

[14] One grins at Pius XI's "moral ruin" of the 1930s. What would he have thought about *Hustler* in corner stores, hardcore pornography that's one click away online, abortion on demand, the institution of "gay" marriage in so many countries, no fault divorce, and condoms in schools?

for the conclusions of *Humanae Vitae*, yet the most combative word he used was "illicit"!

Beneath the diversity of tone, however, is a deeper unity of truth. All popes that have addressed the issue of artificial birth control have spoken with one voice: It is a violation of the pro-life, pro-fecund law God has inscribed in our natures.

Law as Grace and Guide

In its section on the moral life, the *Catechism* is redolent of John Paul II: "Freedom makes man a moral subject. When he acts deliberately, man is, so to speak, *the father of his acts*" (CCC 1749, emphasis in original). Extending this conjugal metaphor, we can say that when we act wisely and well, we give birth within ourselves to twins: happiness and holiness. Following the Lord then becomes an adventure as sweet as it is bracing, because we know that His laws are for our good. As we progress in the Christian life, our salt gets saltier and our light switches more easily to high beam (see Luke 11:36).

With the exception of keeping the Sabbath holy, God did not technically need to reveal the Ten Commandments. But like an accommodating father, He wanted His law to suffuse our darkened minds and weakened wills. As Augustine wrote, "He wrote on the tables of the Law what men did not read in their hearts." With the coming of Christ and the sending of the Holy Spirit, we have an even greater advantage: our searching for God opens our eyes to His search for us and the communication of His loving plan. Unlike, say, the pygmies in Papua or the pagans in pre-Christian Rome, we can't plead invincible ignorance.

Both the Old Law of Moses and the natural law discovered by reason are perfected by the New Law of Christ. This New Law "*is the grace of the Holy Spirit* given to the faithful through faith in Christ. It works through charity; it uses the Sermon on the Mount to teach us what must be done and makes use of the sacraments to give us the grace to do it" (CCC 1966, emphasis in original). It's an inside job, and was already anticipated by the Prophet Jeremiah: "I will make a new covenant with the house of Israel . . . will put my law within them, and I will write it upon their hearts; and I will be their God, and they shall be my people" (Jer 31:31, 33).

As long as we view our response to Christ's covenant as one big inconvenience, we'll never make His will our preference, our first love. As long as our theme song is Sinatra's *My Way*, we'll always balk at doing the right thing. Cardinal Newman called conscience "the connecting principle between the creature and his Creator." In light of our baptism, how much closer does the conscience of children connect them with their doting Father?

The Lord Jesus wants to stay "nickname close" to us as our Best Friend; this is the closeness we need to preserve with Him. "If God is for us, who is against us?" (Rom 8:31). When Baptist leader James MacDonald uses the phrase, "When God says, 'Don't,' he means, 'Don't hurt yourself,'" he lays hold of a very Catholic principle.

Come Lord Jesus, fill me with a newfound love of your law, written naturally in my heart, supernaturally in the Old Law, yet more abundantly in the outpouring of the Spirit of the New. Help me to see your law as my trusted Guide and Rescuer, especially when it comes to the great gift of my sexual desire. I trust in your present and future care for me. Please forgive the ways I have seen your law as my enemy, and grant me the grace to know to love only what is lovely in your sight. Amen.

Chapter Seven

ANSWERS TO THE POP QUIZ

The whole truth is generally the ally of virtue; a half-truth is always the ally of some vice.
—G. K. Chesterton

1. Protestants have always accepted contraception: FALSE. No Protestant body accepted contraception until 1930, when the Anglican bishops, meeting at their Lambeth Conference of that year, overturned all previous Lambeth pronouncements to make a narrow exception to the historic Christian teaching, allowing married couples—for "extraordinary reasons"—to practice birth control. Five hundred years earlier, the Protestant Reformers to a man thundered against all forms of birth control in words more vehement than any pope's. Today, a growing number of Protestants are rediscovering their historic roots.[1]

---

[1] The early Reformers, with no exception, were staunchly anti-birth control. A partial list of Reformation figures and their followers who led the charge includes Martin Luther, John Calvin, John Wesley, Charles Spurgeon, A. W. Pink, Cotton Mather, Matthew Henry, and Adam Clark. Contemporary non-Catholic opponents of contraception include Allan Carlson, PhD, Pastor Matthew Trewhella, Charles

2. *Mahatma Gandhi approved of contraception*: FALSE. The Hindu leader, particularly in the last half of his life, fought strenuously against the introduction of birth control into Indian society. "It is an insult to the fair sex to put up her case in support of birth control by artificial methods," Gandhi wrote. "As it is, man has sufficiently degraded her for his lust, and artificial methods, no matter how well meaning the advocates may be, will still further degrade her. I urge the advocates of artificial methods to consider the consequences. Any large use of the methods is likely to result in the dissolution of the marriage bond and in free love. Birth control to me is a dismal abyss."[2]

3. *Sigmund Freud approved of contraception*. FALSE. The atheist founder of modern psychoanalysis was no bosom buddy of the Catholic Church, yet he viewed birth control as the prime enabler of sexual perversion. Freud wrote that "it is a characteristic common to all the perversions that in them reproduction as an aim is put aside. This is actually the criterion by which we judge whether a sexual activity is perverse—if it departs from reproduction in its aims and pursues the attainment of gratification independently . . . Everything that . . . serves the pursuit of gratification alone is called by the unhonored title of 'perversion' and as such is despised."[3]

D. Provan, Rick and Jan Hess, Ingrid Trobisch, Royce Dunn, Nancy Campbell, Nancy Leigh DeMoss, Mary Pride, and the Quiverfull movement (see www.quiverfull.com).

[2] Quoted by Daniel Vitz in "Gandhi: What He Believed about Sex, Marriage, and Birth Control," *GodSpy*, http://oldarchive.godspy.com/life/Gandhi-on-Sex-Marriage-and-Birth-Control-by-Daniel-Vitz.cfm.html (accessed April 16, 2008).

[3] Sigmund Freud, *A General Introduction to Psycho-Analysis,* translated by Joan Riviere (New York: Liveright, 1935), 277, cited in Donald DeMarco, PhD, "Contraception and Catholic Teaching," http://www.catholic.net/RCC/Periodicals/Faith/11-12-98/Morality2.html.

ANSWERS TO THE POP QUIZ

4. Contraceptives have always been legal in the United States: FALSE. The legislative architect of American anti-contraceptionism was a devout Protestant crusader named Anthony Comstock, whose 1873 Comstock Act forbade the sale and distribution of obscene materials as well as birth control apparatus. These laws were passed in the context of a United States that was mostly Protestant. The last legal battle over public dissemination (no pun intended) of birth control was not fought until 1965, with the US Supreme Court decision *Griswold v. Connecticut.*

Estelle Griswold was a Planned Parenthood director who, along with a Planned Parenthood physician, was convicted as an accessory for giving married couples information and medical advice on how to prevent conception and for prescribing a contraceptive for the wife's use. A Connecticut statute made it a crime for any person to use any drug or article to prevent conception. Griswold and company opened a clinic to test the law, and the challenge went all the way to the US Supreme Court, the majority of which alleged that the "right to privacy" was found implicitly in the Constitution and the Bill of Rights (see next question). The path was made smooth for the *Roe v. Wade* decision eight years later.

5. More contraception leads to fewer abortions: FALSE. On the face of it, it seems very plausible that encouraging "protected" sex will reduce the number of abortions, and many people—anti-abortion and pro-abortion alike—accept this argument. But this reasoning is fallacious. First, the choice to contracept and the choice to abort both stem from the same root: the intention to separate sex from its natural outcome, whether before or after conception. A culture that accepts contraception produces a new need for abortion as a back-up plan in case of an "unwanted pregnancy." Birth control is like stepping out on a high wire. It's fun and exciting, and the crowd roars its approval. Yet you know there's a danger involved. What sane person would start out along that wire without a secure safety net below? That net is abortion.

Put another way, contraception introduces to an act of sexual intercourse an element of negation designed to thwart the coming to be of a baby prior to conception; abortion is the next link in the logical chain: the total negation of a baby already conceived.[4]

The second flaw in the theory is that it ignores the most immediate and obvious effect of birth control: It has, and always will, increase the pool of sexually active people. Since all people naturally desire sex, the availability of birth control has removed one of life's healthy fears: the fear of pregnancy. Birth control has led to a false sense of security by which hundreds of millions of couples now engage in intercourse before or outside wedlock. And since no birth control is foolproof, an additional step was made necessary to "deal with" the "mistake" made with one's sex partner(s). In every country where contraceptive use was widely promoted (late 1960s onward), a corresponding rise in abortions followed.[5]

---

[4] This does not assume that souls pre-exist, waiting around up in heaven somewhere to be born. Contraception does not kill a soul for the simple reason that there is no soul to kill. Yet contraception does interrupt the natural process of sexual union and its procreative power, and it does tamper with the future lives and destinies of our progeny. If two groups of one hundred fertile couples are tracked for five years, one group using birth control, the other using NFP if they have a serious reason to delay pregnancy (i.e., they live a truly Catholic married life), the first group, at the end of five years, would have fewer children than the second. These "missing" children would have been, but are not.

[5] Donald DeMarco, PhD, cites numerous sociological studies that verify this in *New Perspectives on Contraception* (Dayton, OH: One

ANSWERS TO THE POP QUIZ

The line between the end of birth control and the beginning of abortion has already been blurred. And this is not arcane Catholic dogma; it's the solemn opinion of the US Supreme Court. In *Planned Parenthood v. Casey* (505 US 833), the 1992 decision that confirmed *Roe v. Wade* (which legalized abortion at all stages of fetal life), we are told that "in some critical respects, abortion is of the same character as the decision to use contraception . . . for two decades of economic and social developments, people have organized intimate relationships and made choices that define their views of themselves and their places in society, in reliance on the availability of abortion in the event that contraception should fail."

The following dialogue is taken from the transcript of the 1989 Supreme Court decision *Webster v. Reproductive Health Services* (492 US 490). It is highly instructive, considering that the attorney here, Frank Susman, is advocating for the abortion industry (italics mine):

> **Mr. Susman:** For better or worse, *there no longer exists any bright line between the fundamental right that was established in Griswold and the fundamental right of abortion that was established in Roe.* These two rights, because of advances in medicine and science, now overlap. They coalesce and merge and they are not distinct.
>
> **Justice Scalia:** Excuse me, you find it hard to draw a line between those two but easy to draw a line between (the) first, second and third trimester.

More Soul, 1999), 63–73. See also John Noonan, Jr., *Contraception: A History of Its Treatment by the Catholic Theologians and Canonists* (New York: American Library, 1965), 614.

Mr. Susman: I do not find it difficult—

Justice Scalia: I don't see why a court that can draw that line can't separate abortion from birth control quite readily.

Mr. Susman: If I may suggest the reasons in response to your question, Justice Scalia. The most common forms of what we most generally in common parlance call contraception today, IUD's, low-dose birth control pills, which are the safest type of birth control pills available, act as abortifacients. They are correctly labeled as both. *Under this statute, which defines fertilization as the point of beginning, those forms of contraception are also abortifacients.*

Science and medicine refers to them as both. We are not still dealing with the common barrier methods of Griswold. We are no longer just talking about condoms and diaphragms. Things have changed. The bright line, if there ever was one, has now been extinguished.

6. One can be a faithful Catholic and still contracept in good conscience: FALSE. While this stance has gained a wide following after Vatican II (a stance not supported by its documents), the condemnation of contraception is one of the most consistently, authoritatively, and universally taught doctrines by popes (and bishops in union with them), councils, and faithful theologians. See also Number 12 below.

While the Church allows some latitude among scholars engaged in high-level investigation to temporarily withhold public assent to certain positions, this is not what people mean by dissent today, which is some variation of "I want

ANSWERS TO THE POP QUIZ

to do what I want to do despite the teaching." Commenting on this contemporary meaning, the late moral theologian Monsignor William B. Smith noted that the word "dissent" doesn't appear in Catholic encyclopedias until 1972.[6]

This book does not examine the question of whether what is taught in *Humanae Vitae* (if not the encyclical itself) is infallible. I am thoroughly persuaded that it is, and that theologians who argue so are correct.[7] A future pontiff may explicate this, but for now it's a moot point. A given teaching does not need to be formally defined as infallible nor proclaimed by an extraordinary *ex cathedra* statement, such as the Assumption of Mary dogma in 1950 by Pope Pius XI, to merit acceptance by Catholics.

Vatican II clarified that the threshold for assent is not a "sky high" level of formal definition:

> Bishops, teaching in communion with the Roman Pontiff, are to be respected by all as witnesses to divine and Catholic truth. In matters of faith and morals, the bishops speak in the name of Christ and the faithful are to accept their teaching and adhere to it with a religious assent. This religious submission of mind and will must be shown in a special way to the

---

[6] William B. Smith, "The Question of Dissent in Moral Theology," *Persona, Verita, e Morale: Atti del Congresso Internazionale di Teologia Morale* (Roma: Città Nuova Editrice, 1987), 233.

[7] See John Kippley, *Sex and the Marriage Covenant: A Basis for Morality* (Cincinnati, OH: Couple to Couple League, 1991), 159–169; Brian W. Harrison, OS, "*Humanae Vitae* and Infallibility," in *Fidelity* (November 1987), 43–48; a work in Italian by Ermenegildo Lio, OFM, *Humanae Vitae e Infallibilita: il Concilio, Paolo VI e Giovanni Paolo II* (Vatican City: Libreria Editrice Vaticana, 1986); and John C. Ford, SJ, and Germain Grisez, "Contraception and the Infallibility of the Ordinary Magisterium," in *Theological Studies*, vol. 39, no. 2 (June 1978): 258–312.

authentic magisterium of the Roman Pontiff, even when he is not speaking ex cathedra; that is, it must be shown in such a way that his supreme magisterium is acknowledged with reverence, the judgments made by him are sincerely adhered to, according to his manifest mind and will. His mind and will in the matter may be known either from the character of the documents, from his frequent repetition of the same doctrine, or from his manner of speaking.[8]

We must act according to our conscience, yes—our properly formed conscience. What is an unformed conscience but one more human opinion? Again, Vatican II teaches:

> In the formation of their consciences, the Christian faithful ought carefully to attend to the sacred and certain doctrine of the Church. For the Church is, by the will of Christ, the teacher of the truth. It is her duty to give utterance to, and authoritatively to teach, that truth which is Christ Himself, and also to declare and confirm by her authority those principles of the moral order which have their origins in human nature itself. (*DH* 14)

If "faithful Catholic" is to have any meaning, it must involve the duty to form one's mind and heart in light of the Gospel. Even though in some parts of the world there is confusion, the norms of *Humanae Vitae* have never been in doubt by those charged with promulgating the fullness of this Gospel.

---

[8] Second Vatican Council, Dogmatic Constitution on the Church *Lumen Gentium* (November 21, 1964), § 25.

ANSWERS TO THE POP QUIZ

7. The Pill is now medically safe for women: FALSE. Although risks vary, many dangerous or otherwise undesirable side effects of the combination birth control pill and the progestin-only "mini-pill" have been medically established. These include: blood clots, high blood pressure, breast and cervical cancer, liver tumors, migraine headaches, depression, weight gain or loss, and PMS symptoms.[9]

8. The Rhythm Method is now called Natural Family Planning: FALSE. The Rhythm Method was the name of the calendar-based method of family planning discovered simultaneously (and independently) in the 1920s by two gynecologists, Hermann Knaus, MD, of Austria, and Kyusaku Ogino, MD, of Japan. Ironically, Dr. Ogino used his discovery to help infertile women achieve pregnancy. Ogino and Knaus independently discovered that ovulation occurs about fourteen days before the next menstrual period. Abstinence would be gauged by a calendar estimate of infertility. Natural family planning (or NFP for short) refers to several different modern methods of fertility awareness, such as the Ovulation Method, the Sympto-Thermal Method, the Creighton Model, all of which enable, when used correctly, very high rates of effectiveness (97–99 percent).[10] Broadly speaking, NFP methods are based on the daily tracking of biological markers, or signs, of fertility, such as the viscosity (the quality of stick-

---

[9] For a detailed collection of medical evidence, see Paul Weckenbrock, RPh, "The Pill: How Does It Work? Is It Safe?," The Couple to Couple League, http://www.ccli.org/nfp/contraception/pill.phd.

[10] The success rates of properly utilized NFP methods for obtaining or postponing pregnancy are roughly the same. For a comparison between the Billings Ovulations Method and various artificial means, and for an informative breakdown of the financial differences, see Mercedes Urzu Wilson, *Love & Family: How to Raise a Traditional Family in a Secular World* (San Francisco, CA: Ignatius Press, 1996), 246–256.

iness or slipperiness) of cervical mucus and/or the position of the cervix, the presence of breast milk, and the woman's basal body temperature. Comparing these modern methods with Rhythm is like comparing the Wright brothers' rickety glider with a modern jet.

9. The Church teaches that women should have as many babies as possible: FALSE. The Church has never commanded families to propagate into poverty. What the Church teaches is the ideal of generosity when it comes to stewardship of the gift of fertility. The majority of couples today automatically assume that having three—or, horrors, more—children is imprudent and somehow threatening to the well-being of the already-born kids. Encouraging generosity is not the same as mandating numerical quotas. To a culture that aims for small or very small families, the message of generosity does not always sit well.

Stewardship is "in" these days, especially when it comes to writing checks for churchy things. What about stewardship of the power to parenthood? Are buildings, which will one day be dust, more worthy than babies of our "time, talent, and treasure"?

10. The Catholic Church is opposed to all forms of birth regulation: FALSE. Natural family planning, properly understood, involves the regulation of births. As we'll see in Chapter Ten, the difference is that regulation is not repudiation. In his book *The Well and the Shadows*, G. K. Chesterton noted, "What is quaintly called Birth Control . . . is in fact, of course, a scheme for preventing birth in order to escape control." With NFP, the couple exercises their gift of fertility in partnership with God, always leaving the baby-blessing trump card in His hands. But with contraception, God's special participation is shunned altogether.

11. The Bible does not mention contraception: FALSE. See Chapter Four.

12. Catholic teaching against contraception is fixed and cannot change: TRUE. The teaching belongs to the deposit of the Catholic faith. Whenever the Catholic position has been attacked, as historian John Noonan notes, "the teachers of the Church have taught without hesitation or variation that certain acts preventing procreation are gravely sinful. No Catholic theologian has ever taught, 'contraception is a good act.' The teaching is clear and apparently fixed forever."[11] Contrary to the fantasies of its foes, the teaching is normative for all times, an ineluctable, irreformable part of Catholicism. As St. Pope John Paul II told the 1988 Moral Theology Congress in Rome, "By describing the contraceptive act as intrinsically illicit, Paul VI meant to teach that the moral norm is such that it does not admit exceptions. No personal or social circumstance could ever, can now, or will ever, render such an act lawful in itself." In other words, the wrongness of contraception is not due to arbitrary or "sectarian" decree, but to the very moral structure of human nature in its capacity to bring forth new life. The Church can no easier proclaim black to be white.

This last question was the reef against which my own ship of dissent capsized, as mentioned in Chapter Two. There is little reason to accept the Resurrection if for two thousand years the Church could teach something so cataclysmically

---

[11] Noonan, *Contraception*, xix.

false and misleading to hundreds of millions of couples. If what *Humanae Vitae* teaches is false, then Catholicism is a false religion—a conclusion that at least has consistency on its side.

If you peel away all of life's nuances and subtleties, the intellectual flotsam and jetsam of rationalizations to which human nature is inclined, life comes down ultimately to only two alternatives: "either one conforms desire to the truth or one conforms truth to desire."[12]

The question of Jesus to His apostles, "Who do you say that I am?" (Matt 16:15), rings down through the centuries to our ears. Simon Peter got the answer right in his time. Answering it rightly, and living by it, is our task in ours.

---

[12] E. Michael Jones, *Degenerate Moderns: Modernity As Rationalized Sexual Misbehavior* (San Francisco, CA: Ignatius Press, 1993), 11.

Chapter Eight

THE POPULATION BOMB MYTH
An Answer to Chicken Little

Too many children? That's like saying, "Too many flowers."
—Saint Mother Teresa of Calcutta

A *New Yorker* cartoon shows a toddler standing in the doorway of his parents' bedroom. He says, "I've had another bad dream about Social Security." We chuckle, but the little guy spoke more demographic truth than the cartoonist likely intended.

The belief that the world is overpopulated—or soon will be—has a lot going for it. Except that it isn't true.

While the question of whether the earth does or does not face a population explosion has nothing to do with the wrongness of contraception, it's a myth worth exploding. For few debates over birth control get very far before Uncle Tom, co-worker Dick, or Professor Harry will bring up the "population explosion" problem and why birth control is part of the solution. Those who promote the "There Are Too

Many of Us Already" propaganda are very up front about what they mean: (a) we must slow down the arrival speed of new babies (the domain of contraception and abortion); and (b) we must speed up their exit (the domain of suicide and euthanasia). Both "solutions" are alive and well, and gaining traction and respectability everywhere.

The population explosion scare is almost universally assumed to be an accurate assessment of humanity's alleged predicament (shades of former Vice President Gore's assertion that the debate about global warming is "over"). This chapter will show that earthlings do face a population crisis: a population implosion.

Not only have most people not heard this information, there is probably as much resistance to it as there is to the Church's opposition to birth control itself. We will now browse the history of the overpopulation movement, review some fascinating demographic projections for the future, and provide some facts with which to explode the myth of overpopulation.

We Have Met the Enemy and It Wears Diapers, Naps a Lot

While there are a few references to the perceived need to prune overpopulation in ancient Greece,[1] the modern overpopulation bandwagon picked up speed in the year 1798 with the publication of *An Essay on the Principle of Popu-*

---

[1] The plot lines of some Greek myths reflected current events and concerns. There is a reference to overpopulation in *The Cypria*, a part of the Epic cycle that, along with Homer's Iliad and Odyssey, relates the history of the Trojan War, by which Zeus was moved to prune population levels. There are also expressions of worry over a population explosion in Confucius and Plato, as well as in the work of early Christian writers Tertullian and St. Jerome.

lation, by an Anglican clergyman and economist named Thomas Malthus. The ideas contained in this work attracted many admirers, one of the earliest being Charles Darwin. Reverend Malthus's argument boiled down to a simple proposition: The world's food production grows arithmetically (1, 2, 3, 4, 5 . . .) but its population rate grows exponentially (1, 2, 4, 8, 16 . . .). Thus sooner or later, he argued, the human race would encounter the world's scariest math: Too many mouths + too few carrots = inevitable mass death by starvation.

Malthus was convinced that overpopulation caused poverty, disease, and war, and that all social remedies were doomed to fail unless the torrent of new children into the world could be halted for a time. It may be true that overpopulation could have occurred already if it weren't for famines, pandemics, wars, natural disasters, historically high rates of infant death, celibate clergy, and the like. But as Dr. Halliday Sutherland wrote in 1920s England:

> The truth of these facts is indisputable, but it is a manifest breach of logic to argue from the fact of poverty, disease and war having checked an increase in population, that therefore poverty, disease and war are due to an increase of population. It would be as reasonable to argue that, because an unlimited increase of insects is prevented by birds and by climatic changes, therefore an increase of insects accounts for the existence of birds and climatic changes.[2]

---

[2] Halliday G. Sutherland, MD, *Birth Control: A Statement of Christian Doctrine against the Neo-Malthusians* (Whitefish, MT: Kessinger Publishing, 2004), 7. Originally published by P.J. Kennedy in New York, 1922.

Reverend Malthus argued that there were two main ways to avert the coming disaster: by exercising moral restraint through abstinence, or by indulging in vice. (Christians living in pre-Lambeth England understood vice to mean contraception.) While Malthus was not wrong in his predictions of population growth, his food catastrophe never arrived. Famines have, indeed, appeared in certain areas for certain periods since then, and the horrible phenomenon of starvation still exists in some parts of the world. But the rise of agricultural technology and the development of new ways to produce and distribute high-quality foods, and the unforeseen decline of birth rates since the mid-twentieth century, have sharply contradicted his dire predictions.

Among Malthus's latter day protégés, the most famous is American biologist Dr. Paul Ehrlich. His book *The Population Bomb*, which appeared the same year as *Humanae Vitae*, is a bible of 1960s enthusiasms. In it, he rails against US hegemony and imperialism, the pesticide DDT, corporate greed, and proffers feverish arguments on behalf of federal laws requiring explicit sex education in public schools prior to junior high school. As you would expect, Ehrlich stridently promoted an unlimited abortion license, which came down five years after his book came out.

The Population Bomb is nothing if not earnest in its pessimism—think Chicken Little with a PhD and a bullhorn. It's remarkable that a book with so many accidentally hilarious predictions would remain so influential. It opens with this gem: "The battle to feed all of humanity is over. In the 1970s and 1980s, hundreds of millions of people will starve to death, in spite of any crash programs embarked upon now."[3]

---

[3] Paul Ehrlich, PhD, *The Population Explosion* (New York: Ballantine Books, 1968), Prologue.

How tenderly Dr. Ehrlich regards his fellow human beings: "A cancer is an uncontrolled multiplication of cells; the population explosion is an uncontrolled multiplication of people. . . . We must shift our efforts from treatment of the symptoms to the cutting out of the cancer. The operation will demand many apparently brutal and heartless decisions. The pain may be intense. But the disease is so far advanced that only with radical surgery does the patient have a chance of survival."[4]

Ehrlich the theory, Hitler the practice.

Today, the fear of overpopulation has saturated the public imagination. Its unspoken endgame scenario is like a Hollywood disaster movie featuring millions of people crowded together on tip toe along the coasts and around lakes, angling not to fall into the water; pandemics brought on by massive malnutrition, civil wars over food rations, and masses of urban refugees fleeing into ever-crowded desert regions. Unless "something" is "done" "soon," Montana will one day wake up as Manhattan. Or something like that.

I jest, but only partly, for this line of thinking has been granted sacred cow status by school and college textbooks, and is echoed by almost every media outlet.[5] (It has a cousin, too: the ubiquitous evolution tableaux in which a tadpole becomes a fish, a lizard, an ape, a caveman, and then upright homo sapiens, as if Darwinian theory is 100 percent correct.)

This new orthodoxy defines the goals of many inter-related political organizations such as Planned Parenthood, the

---

[4] Ehlrich, *The Population Explosion,* 152.
[5] For a comprehensive catalogue of government-funded educational programs that rely on these presuppositions, see Jacqueline Kasun, PhD, *The War against Population: The Economics and Ideology of World Population Control* (San Francisco, CA: Ignatius Press, 1999), 25–34.

Population Institute, the Sierra Club, The National Abortion Rights Action League (NARAL), the Ford and Rockefeller Foundations, and Zero Population Growth (ZPG).[6] Few myths have friends in such high places: efforts at halting the spread of wretched humanity have been the official policy of the United States since the Administration of President Lyndon B. Johnson.[7]

If you have no idea it's a scam, or at best a mistaken theory, the fear is easy enough to buy into. However, if old age homes start outnumbering nurseries, and casket sales outstrip those of cradles, then the human race would indeed be on a collision course with disaster.

Night of the Living Birth Dearth

Birthrates around the world are falling steadily and, in many industrialized countries such as Great Britain and most of Europe, have been doing so since the end of World War II. Demographer Ben Wattenberg wrote about this in his 1987 book *The Birth Dearth* and, more recently, in *Fewer: How the New Demography of De-Population Will Shape Our Future*. He notes:

> For the last 650 years, since the time of the Black Plague, the total number of people on earth has headed in only one direction: up. But soon—prob-

---

[6] Two new books explore this trend and its history. See Steven Mosher, *Population Control: Real Costs, Illusory Benefits* (Edison, NJ: Transaction Publishing, 2008), and Matthew Connelly, *The Struggle to Control World Population* (Harvard University Press/Belknap, 2008).

[7] See, for example, *Population and the American Future: The Report of the Commission on Population Growth and the American Future* (New York: New American Library, 1972), 137, 171, 178, 189–190, cited in Kasun, 219.

ably within a few decades—global population will level off and then likely fall for a protracted period of time. The number of people on earth will be headed down, "depopulating." Why? *Birthrates and fertility rates ultimately yield total population levels. And never have birth and fertility rates fallen so far, so fast, so low, for so long, in so many places, so surprisingly.*[8] (Italics are his.)

Of course, to say that birth rates are falling in most countries is not to deny that the overall population of the world is increasing. It is. The rub is that the rate of new persons being born has already started a vast slowdown. In general, parents in most parts of the world are electing to have fewer and fewer kids.

If that sounds counterintuitive, policy journalist Philip Longman provides an analogy of a train chugging uphill:

> If the engine stalls, the train will still move forward for a while, but its loss of momentum implies that it will soon be moving backwards, and at ever-greater speed. So it is when fertility rates shift from above to below replacement levels. The equivalent of the hill is death itself, which is always pushing against any increase in human population. The equivalent of the engine is a fertility rate that consistently produces more births than deaths ... specifically, when women born during a period of high fertility (such as the 1950s in the United States) wind up having fewer children than their mothers, population size

---

[8] Ben J. Wattenberg, *Fewer: How the New Demography of De-Population Will Shape Our Future* (Chicago: Ivan Dee Publishing, 2004), 5.

may well still grow because of the large number of women of childbearing age. But in the next generation, the pool of potential mothers will be smaller than before, and in the generation after that, the pool become smaller still. By then the momentum of population growth is lost, or more precisely, is working in the opposite direction with compounding force.[9]

And what is that magic fertility replacement rate? It's 2.1 children, a statistical way of saying that a human population base can only maintain its current level over an extended time if each set of parents have two kids to replace themselves, plus "more." (The 0.1 accounts for infant mortality and for offspring who die before childbearing age.) There will always be people who stay single, couples with no children, and couples with van-loads of children, but the population must maintain an average family size of slightly more than two children to sustain the replacement level.

Since the 1950s, when five- and six-kid families were commonplace (a fact well known to anyone who was an adult at the time), the average family size has dropped dramatically.[10] The anecdotal evidence of this drop is everywhere. Today's ideal is two kids, preferably a boy and a girl because that's so cute. In magazines, on billboards, and on television, advertisers spend millions of dollars projecting the two-child family as the image of choice.

---

[9] Philip Longman, *The Empty Cradle: How Falling Birthrates Threaten World Prosperity and What to Do about It* (New York: Basic Books, 2004), 12.

[10] In the award-winning 1950 comedy *Cheaper by the Dozen*, based on the true-life Gilbreth family, Clifton Webb played the efficiency engineer father of twelve. At one point, he sniffles at "those piddly little families with only five or six children." The scene where the Planned Parenthood lady pays a visit (and is hilariously rebuffed) was, unsurprisingly, cut from the 2003 remake starring Steve Martin.

THE POPULATION BOMB MYTH

17 FAST FACTS

In the United States, Canada, and most of Europe, young parents violate an unwritten taboo when they have a third or fourth child, drawing the gossipy stares and *tsk-tsks* of those whom one perceptive mom has called "the fertility police."[11] Usually it's in the form of well-meant ribbing ("Hey, do you guys know what you're doing?" "They have pills for that, you know," and so on), but the barbs can be downright rude. Why is it anyone's business? Parents might ask the joker, "Which of my kids would the world be better without?"

I will close this chapter with some facts arranged in cheat sheet form. Commit a few of them to memory so you can give Tom, Dick, or Harry something to think about the next time they invoke the population explosion myth as a way of excusing contraception:

Fact 1: One of the easiest ways to disprove that the earth is anywhere near being overpopulated is to get in an airplane and take off from any of the world's largest cities: Beijing, New York, Tokyo, New Delhi, London, Paris, Shanghai, Mexico City, or Toronto. After fifteen minutes in the air, look down. You will see mostly green vistas, smooth plains, rivers, and rolling hills.

Fact 2: World population growth is slowing down at an alarming rate. United Nations figures show that the seventy-nine countries that make up 40 percent of the world's population now have fertility rates well below replacement level.

---

[11] Mary Walsh, "Wanted by the Fertility Police," in *Family Foundations*, a publication of The Couple to Couple League, accessed from www.ccli.org. See resources Appendix.

Fact 3: 46 percent of the earth is still pristine wilderness, undeveloped, and nearly unpopulated. This area, roughly sixty-eight million square miles, is home to only 2.4 percent of the world's population.[12]

Fact 4: The population of the entire world, at the printing of this book, could fit into the State of Texas with each person living on almost a third of an acre.[13] This fact alone disproves the image of the earth's surface brimming with sardine-like humanity. (See Fact 16.)

Fact 5: Africa is often held up as incontrovertible evidence that overpopulation causes poverty, or, according to the opposite theory, is caused by poverty. But Africa has only one-fifth the population density of Europe. According to estimates by Roger Revelle, former director of the Harvard Center for Population Studies, and research by the University of California at San Diego, the continent of Africa has an unexploited agricultural capacity to feed twice the present population of the world.[14]

Fact 6: A 2005 Statistics Canada study, describing Canada's population plunge as an "unprecedented situation," revealed

---

[12] This does not include oceans and lakes, according to an intensive two-year study by Conservation International. See Paul Rogers, "46 Percent of Earth is Still Wilderness, Researchers Report," *The Mercury News*, Dec. 4, 2002.

[13] See http://www.ibiblio.org/lunarbin/worldpop for an approximate running tab of the world's population. Divide this total number into the size of Texas, which is 268,601 square miles (http://www.netstate.com/states/geography/tx_geography.htm) and you get 0.27 acres per earthling.

[14] Dr. Jacqueline R. Kasun, "Too Many People?" in *Envoy Magazine*, May–June 1998, accessible online at http://www.envoymagazine.com/backissues/2.3/coverstory.html.

that Canada is aging so fast that senior citizens over sixty-five will outnumber children under fifteen a decade from now.[15]

Fact 7: Japan recently experienced its first ever drop in overall population owing to its very low 1.3 fertility level, as 70 percent of young Japanese women now report having no interest in marrying. In the last decade, ninety theme parks for children in Japan have disappeared, and several thousand elementary schools and pediatric hospitals have closed.[16]

Fact 8: While all the European nations' birthrates have spiraled dramatically down, the German Federal Statistics Office reports that Germany has remained below the replacement fertility rate (1.36) for so long that it has reached the point of no return, a situation that can no longer be countered by immigration.[17]

Fact 9: Russia's population drops by almost 750,000 people yearly. President Vladimir Putin has called Russia's birth dearth "the most acute problem facing the country."[18] Attempts at a remedy have included cash incentives for having more than one child (as is done in Quebec), special pensions for extra fertile mothers, and the Day of Concep-

---

[15] LifeSiteNews.com, "Canada in Population Crisis: Seniors to Outnumber Children in a Decade," December 15, 2005, http://www.lifesite.net/ldn/2005/dec/05121504.html (accessed August, 2007).

[16] "A Baby Bust Empties Out Japan's Schools: Shrinking Population Called Greatest National Problem" by Anthony Faiola in *The Washington Post Foreign Service*, March 3, 2005, A01.

[17] Report from Deutsche Welle, Berlin, November 9, 2006, as reported by Gudrun Schultz in *Lifesite News*, accessed August 2007 from http://www.lifesite.net/ldn/2006/nov/06110903.html.

[18] United Nations Population Division, "Replacement Migration: Is It a Solution to Declining and Aging Populations?" (2000), cited in Longman, 60.

tion, held annually on September 12 in the Ulyanovsk region. The contest provides a day off for patriotic couples to do what comes naturally—in order to win cash prizes, refrigerators, and SUVs.[19] I kid you not.

Fact 10: By 1900, Russian women bore an average of seven children over a lifetime. At the collapse of the Soviet Union, this had dropped to 1.7.

Fact 11: The US military budget provides a surprising benchmark of how the American population at large is aging. In 2000, the cost of military pensions amounted to twelve times what the Pentagon spent on ammunition; nearly five times what the Navy spent on new warships, and over five times what the Air Force spent on new planes and missiles.[20]

Fact 12: Many of the world's most densely populated areas also happen to provide high levels of per capita wealth and economic stability, such as The Netherlands, Japan, Singapore, Taiwan, and Hong Kong. South Korea's population density is 3.6 times higher than China's, yet boasts a per capita output twelve times greater.[21]

---

[19] Sometimes, real news mimics Onion-style news parodies, e.g., "Russia's Conception Day: Have a June Baby, Win a Prize," by Liza Kuznetsova, *The Associated Press,* August 15, 2007.

[20] Office of the Under Secretary of Defense (Comptroller), *Department of Defense Budget Fiscal Years 2004/2005: Military Personnel Programs (M-1)* (February 2003), 22, http://www.dod.mil/comptroller/defbudget/fy2004_m1.pdf, cited in Longman, 21.

[21] Julian L. Simon and Roy Gobi, "The Relationship between Population and Economic Growth in LDCs," in Julian L. Simon, *Population and Development in Poor Countries: Selected Essays* (Princeton University Press, 1992), 191, cited in Kasun, *The War against Population,* 69–70.

Fact 13: Executive management and economic guru Dr. Peter Drucker, author of over thirty books on economics and business leadership, says, "the most important single new certainty—if only because there is no precedent for it in all of history—is the collapsing birthrate in the developed world."[22]

Fact 14: George Orwell said that some ideas are so dumb that only an intellectual could believe them. Lizard expert and ecologist Dr. Eric Pianka is an intellectual. The University of Texas at Austin professor believes that the population of the earth could stand a 90 percent reduction, and has publicly suggested that the deadly airborne Ebola virus would do the trick nicely. "We're no better than bacteria," he opined.[23] (As of this writing, Pianka has still not removed himself from the planet by way of an Ebola cocktail.) Sadly, even the revered oceanographer Jacques Cousteau offered his own unfortunate final solution: "It's terrible to have to say this. World population must be stabilized and to do that we must eliminate 350,000 people per day. This is so horrible to contemplate that we shouldn't even say it. But the general situation in which we are involved is lamentable."[24] These are the public thoughts of the population scare movement.

Fact 15: Despite having a higher average TFR (total fertility rate) than most western countries, the overall fertility rates

---

[22] Peter Drucker, *Management Challenges for the 21st Century* (New York: HarperBusiness, 1999), 44.

[23] Eric R. Pianka, PhD, lecture given at the 109th meeting of the Texas Academy of Science at Lamar University in Beaumont on March 3–5, 2006, as reported in *The Citizen Scientist*, by Forrest Mims III and witnessed by others, http://www.sas.org/tcs/weeklyIssues_2006/2006-04-07/feature1p/index.html.

[24] Interview in *UNESCO Courier*, November, 1991, by Bahgat Elnadi.

in the United States have fallen steadily since 1801, with the exception of the post-World War II baby boom, which peaked in 1957.[25]

Fact 16: Advances in agricultural science have made obsessions over food shortages moot. The Food and Agricultural Association reports that, at present, farmers use less than half of the world's arable land. "The conversion of land to urban and built-up uses to accommodate a larger population will absorb less than 2 percent of the world's land, and 'is not likely to seriously diminish the supply of land for agricultural production,' according to Paul Waggoner, writing for the Council for Agricultural Science and Technology in 1994."[26]

Fact 17: Most people have never thought about where their logic leads them. The next time a Chicken Little in your life plays the overpopulation card, turn it around and ask him how few people on earth would be ideal, and why.

---

[25] Longman, *The Empty Cradle*, 87.
[26] Jacqueline Kasun, "Overpopulation?," *LifeIssues.net*, http://www.lifeissues.net/writers/kas/kas_01overpopulation.html. Then there is the virtually unknown work of Norman Borlaug, Nobel laureate, winner of the Congressional Gold Medal, and the "father of the Green Revolution." His spectacularly successful biotech innovations in wheat and cereal production in India, Pakistan, Africa, Mexico, and elsewhere in the Third World have been credited with saving over a billion lives. See http://www.normanborlaug.org/.

Chapter Nine

PLANNED BARRENHOOD
Sterilization and Its Discontents

A bruised reed he will not break; and a dimly burning wick he will not quench.

—Isaiah 42:3

Sterilization presents a delicate and difficult pastoral challenge for three groups of people: those who wish to share the teaching of the Church; those who've been sterilized and have come to regret it; and those who've been sterilized and do not regret it. The sense of finality that attends the procedure creates a mindset that is not well disposed to second-guessing. The pill and female sterilization have been the two most commonly used methods since 1982, followed by the IUD and male vasectomy.[1]

You can always toss your condoms, jellies, foams, or diaphragms in the trash, or cancel your Pill prescription, but you can't wake up one day and de-sterilize yourself when

---

[1] Daniels K, Daugherty J and Jones J, Current contraceptive status among women aged 15–44: United States, 2011–2013, *National Health Statistics Reports*, 2014, no. 173, http://www.cdc.gov/nchs/data/databriefs/db173.pdf.

you've chosen contraception to the -nth degree. At least not easily. Apart from the option of reversing the sterilization, to be discussed later in this chapter, the quasi-permanent aspect of sterilization can make it very difficult psychologically to even admit that a mistake has been made.

Even if the couple (the sterilized man or woman in the couple) regrets and repents of the procedure—and for whatever reason cannot have the reversal—they may find themselves living in a curious state of limbo in which they continue to "enjoy the fruits of their sin," in the memorable phrase of the Couple to Couple League founder John Kippley.

This chapter will propose some strategies for resolving this dilemma, review the nature and risks involved with male and female sterilization, discuss the marital frictions associated with these procedures, and end with some questions meant to stimulate important conversations between spouses, and to encourage apologists to think outside the "repent, sinner" box.

Someone may ask why I'd bother treating sterilization in depth. Isn't it just a guilt trip to dwell on a sincere decision made perhaps long ago? If they can't do anything about it, what's the point in tormenting them?

Fair questions.

In reflecting on an answer, a Scripture verse said to be a favorite of St. John Paul II came to mind: "You will know the truth, and the truth will make you free" (John 8:32). What can be "done about it" is precisely the theme of this chapter. No one loses his or her right to the truth just because of a mistake made or a sin committed. Ultimately—for every one of us—lies enslave; half-truths hobble. The whole truth frees.

None of this is about finger-pointing. Most people who chose sterilization did what they thought was the right thing to do, and did it without malice toward the Church. They didn't wake up in the morning and ask themselves what's the best way to offend God or defy the Church. Indeed, many are active in parish life. In the main, they were never told otherwise about sterilization, or a Church representative validated their decision, or they had the procedure before they became Catholic.

The combination of silence from the pulpit and the great acceptance of sterilization fostered by society (by the medical profession in particular)[2] give it a very attractive luster. Minus the support of knowledgeable Catholic friends and family, the seeming benefits of sterilization—its one-shot-and-you're-done convenience, its permanence, and its user effectiveness—have made it the most popular form of contraception.[3] Well-intentioned bromides provide added incentive and validation ("It's okay as long as you have good intentions." . . . "Vatican II says we must follow our conscience." . . . "God understands our weaknesses." . . . "You've already been generous enough by having X number of kids.").

It's a simple fact: Most people simply have never heard a rational explanation why sterilization could be immoral.

Defining the Thing

Sterilization refers to any surgical procedure that is intended to deliberately and permanently render a man or a woman

---

[2] In Canada, all forms of sterilization are covered by its free (sic) universal health care system. Most US insurance companies cover vasectomies and tubal ligations. Invariably, reversals are not covered under either system.

[3] Its effectiveness explains its popularity. Sterilization comes second only to lifelong virginity and chemical castration for certainty of pregnancy prevention. The majority of post-vasectomy pregnancies stem from the couple having intercourse too soon after the procedure.

infertile. The male version is better known as a vasectomy. In a vasectomy, the *vasa deferentia* (two thin tubes that connect the testes to the rest of the reproductive system), are cut and then cauterized or sutured. The sperm become trapped in the testes and are unable to complete their journey toward the ovum, and are then broken down and absorbed into the blood vessels and lymph tissues of the man's body. The body is thus "auto-immune," or allergic to itself. This happens about 88 percent of the time within six months.

The first modern attempts at sterilization had nothing to do with improving family life, advancing healthcare technology, or even with medical care itself. It was done as part of prison experimentations between the 1890s to early 1900s when sterilizing jailed sexual predators became a popular alternative to full castration (removal of the testes).[4]

The moral assessment of sterilization differs only in degree from other kinds of contraception. Given the element of mutilation involved,[5] along with the intention of permanence, all reliable moral theologians teach that sterilization is more seriously wrong than the other methods. While all birth control is on the level of mortal sin, the three conditions for mortal sin—grave matter, full knowledge, and deliberate consent—have not generally been met in the lives of most contracepting couples today, particularly because of a lack in the second condition.[6] As we will see, this does

---

[4] See www.vasectomy-information.com/moreinfo/history.htm (accessed January 18, 2008). These experiments helped launch eugenics laws that allowed for the involuntary sterilization of men, women, and children considered "defective." Over thirty states had such laws.

[5] We are not talking about procedures that transgress healthy tissues en route to repairing or removing diseased organs. But deliberate sterilization is precisely the mutilation of an otherwise healthy organ and is not done for curative reasons.

[6] See CCC 1857.

not mean that the decision will have no ill effects on bodies or marriages. You can innocently walk off a ledge but that doesn't mean the law of gravity won't take its toll on you rather quickly.

Side Effects They Don't Advertise

There is a tendency in the sterilization "information literature" to downplay the possible complications, risks, and negative side effects that can surface down the road. One might object that all surgical procedures entail some element of risk. And that is true. Bad side effects do not always, in themselves, make bad acts. In this case, however, even if medical science one day produced a method of sterilization with absolutely no bad side effects, sterilization would still be gravely immoral. (This is also true of the Pill.)

The absorption of sperm cells following a vasectomy is tied to one of many negative side effects. The man's body interprets the sudden presence of the sperm cells as foreign matter and, to protect itself against the antigens produced by degenerated sperms cells, manufactures antibodies to combat the foreign invaders.

Medical science has known about this phenomenon since the early 1970s, when antibodies generated against sperm antigens were found in 55–75 percent of vasectomized men two years following the procedure.[7] The implications of autoimmune disorders arising from vasectomy are not yet fully known. But some side effects include:

---

[7] J. D. Matthews et al., "Weak Antibody Reactions to Antigens Other than Sperm after Vasectomy," *British Medical Journal* (1976) 2:1359; R. Ansbacher et al., "Sperm Antibodies in Vasectomized Men," *Fertility and Sterility* (1972): 23:640.

- *Pain*: While post-surgery pain should theoretically stop after about a week, some men report irritation and discomfort in the groin years later when riding a bike or sliding across the front car seat.
- *Granulomas*: The leakage of sperm from the snipped vasa into the scrotal tissues can cause benign (non-cancerous) lumps resulting from an inflammatory reaction. These sperm granulomas may be tender to the touch and, more rarely, develop into an abscess.
- *Erectile dysfunction or decreased sexual desire*: This can occur in the form of impotence, premature ejaculation, or painful intercourse, which may be partly psychological in nature. The vasectomy can also exacerbate previous problems between sexual partners.
- *Link to early onset dementia*: Researchers at Northwestern University studied forty-seven men aged fifty-five to eighty with a language-based dementia known as Primary Progressive Aphasia (PPA), and found that 40 percent had had vasectomies, compared to 16 percent of the control group with no cognitive impairment.[8]
- *Cancer*: Studies from the early 1990s have progressively shown an association between vasectomy and

---

[8] Sandra Weintraub, PhD, Marek-Marsel Mesulam, MD, et al., *Cognitive & Behavioral Neurology* 19(4),190–193, (December 2006). Dr. Weintraub is professor of psychiatry at the Feinberg School of Medicine. At a Chicago support group meeting for PPA sufferers, one of her patients polled the men sitting there. "OK, guys, how many of you have PPA?" Nine hands were raised. "And how many of you had a vasectomy?" the man continued. Eight hands shot up. See Marla Paul, "Vasectomy may put men at risk for dementia," *Observer online*, http://www.northwestern.edu/observer/issues/2007/03/28/vasectomy.html (accessed December 13, 2007).

an increased risk of various kinds of cancers, such as lung cancer, non-Hodgkin's lymphoma, and multiple myeloma.[9]

For women, the procedure is similar and is called a tubal ligation, better known as "having your tubes tied." This procedure also entails considerable risks, including:

- *Serious complications at the time of surgery*: Depending on which kind of ligation method chosen, between 800 and 2,000 women per 100,000 can expect a major complication at the time of the procedure, such as infection, injury to the bladder or bleeding from a major blood vessel, burning of the bowel or other neighboring tissues, and anesthesia complications.[10]
- *Increased risk of ectopic pregnancy*: Approximately one half of pregnancies resulting despite the ligation will result in an ectopic pregnancy, a painful and potentially lethal event in which the egg is fertilized and begins to attach and grow outside the uterus, usually in the Fallopian tube.

---

[9] See L. Rosenberg, J. R. Palmer, A. G. Zauber, et al., "Vasectomy and the Risk of Prostate Cancer," *American Journal of Epidemiology* (1990), 132:1051–1055; C. Mettlin, N. Natarajan, and P. Huben, "Vasectomy and prostate cancer risk," *American Journal of Epidemiology* (1990), 132:1056–1061; E. Giovannucci, A. Ascherio, E. B. Rimm, et al., "A Prospective Cohort Study of Vasectomy and Prostate Cancer in U.S. Men," *Journal of the American Medical Association* (1993), 269:873–877; E. Giovanucci, T. D. Tosteson, F. E. Speizer, et al., "A retrospective cohort study of vasectomy and prostate cancer in U. S. men," *Journal of the American Medical Association* (1993), 269:878–882, all cited in Keith Bower, "Vasectomy: Some Questions and Answers," Couple to Couple League, http://www.ccli.org/nfp/contraception/vasectomy.php.

[10] Susan Harlap, Kathryn Kost, and Jacqueline Darroch Forrest, *Preventing Pregnancy, Protecting Health: A New Look at Birth Control Choices in the United States* (New York: Alan Guttmacher Institute, 1991), 92.

- Other lesser known risks include *menstrual irregularities and prolonged bleeding, increased cramping, and post-tubal sterilization syndrome (a form of depression)*.[11]

Getting Unfixed

It is not well known that both vasectomies and TLs (tubal ligations) can be reversed with varying success rates, reckoned as somewhere between fifty to 75 percent.[12] Achieving a post-reversal pregnancy depends mainly on how much time has elapsed since the sterilization, how frequently the physician performs the procedure, and whether the physical structures of the vasa and the Fallopian tubes remain conducive to reattachment.

Although reversal surgeries are more costly and more complicated than sterilization itself, a growing number of people are choosing them. Even if they don't bring another baby into the world, the testimonies of people who changed their minds make for moving and enriching reading. I highly recommend *Sterilization Reversal: A Generous Act of Love*, a unique collection of twenty couples' stories edited by John Long, and a conference talk by David and Nina Morton titled "Testimony of Healing," both available from One More Soul (see Appendix).

---

[11] For a review of the medical literature on the side effects and risks of the TL, see Keith Bower, *Tubal Ligation: Some Questions and Answers*, an educational pamphlet published by the Couple to Couple League, found online at http://www.ccli.org/nfp/contraception/tubal.php.

[12] John L. Long, ed., *Sterilization Reversal: A Generous Act of Love* (Dayton, OH: One More Soul, 2003). For reversal stories from a Pentecostal perspective, see Nancy Campbell, ed., *A Change of Heart* (Franklin, TN: Above Rubies Ministries, 2006). More testimonies from Protestant couples may be found on Marshall's website www.aboverubies.org.

As we saw in Chapter Five, the natural law is inviolable in the sense that flouting its directives eventually brings consequences, and not all of them foreseen. Since man is a union of matter and spirit, some of the side effects associated with vasectomy and tubal ligation may, in fact, be psychosomatic. God doesn't punish arbitrarily the way an office manager might punish a clerk who steals a stapler. Rather, every unnatural act carries with it some repercussion, sooner or later, in this life or the next.

Dr. Gregory Polito, a Southern California urologist who performs vasovasostomies (aka, vasectomy reversals), knows this firsthand. He notes that not nearly enough research has been done to track the long-term repercussions—personal, marital, and social—of sterilization.[13]

In his clinical experience, patients who change their minds and have their vasectomies reversed invariably felt that something was awry but couldn't put their finger on it—at first. "You don't need to bring in a lot of theology," Dr. Polito notes. "They've already detected a problem in their marriage, something 'off,' even apart from the new desire for more kids."[14]

The Long Shadow of Regret

Regardless of religious belief, most reasonable people admit that an operation that intentionally destroys the capacity for fatherhood or motherhood is not the same as operations such as a heart bypass or a kidney transplant. In sterilization, of all the myriad types of cells in the man's body, the only one with a singular role in co-creating new human beings—

---

[13] Gregory Polito, MD, KM, "The Consequences of Vasectomy and Its Reversal," Appendix in *Sterilization Reversal*, 293.
[14] In discussion with author, November 1, 2007.

the sperm cell—is treated as a threat to be (literally) cut out of the picture.

In trading fertility for sterility, each subsequent sex act therefore loses the objective quality of openness to new life required by sacramental marriage. It is "seriously stained," as Kippley puts it.[15] For Catholics, at least, the decision results in an ongoing, implicit violation of their wedding vows when they promised "to welcome children lovingly from God, and bring them up according to the law of Christ and the Church."

As it happens, if one of the spouses comes to regret the decision, they can spend many years hiding their regret.[16] There are no studies extant on how many people change their minds about the procedure, but even if it's a large number, regret doesn't necessarily translate into reversal. Only about 1 percent of vasectomies and TLs are reversed, but that doesn't tell us how many more live with the daily anguish of knowing they made a serious mistake and for whatever reason are unable to correct it.

Everyone reading this book knows firsthand how stubborn human nature can be. As children of Adam, we are allergic to the phrase, "I was wrong." The precinct inhabited by a sterilized person, however, makes this allergy worse. Feeling "locked in," a pattern of self-justification and rationalization can, over time, squelch the voice of conscience that is "inscribed by God in the human heart," in the words of the Second Vatican Council (GS 16).

---

[15] Kippley, *Sex and the Marriage Covenant*, 208.
[16] Dr. Herbert Peterson conducted a long-term study of 10,685 sterilized women aged eighteen to forty-four who were followed from 1978 to 1992. One in five women under age thirty who undergoes tubal sterilization later regrets having the procedure. See also, Nancy Walsh, "A Fifth of Women Regret the Decision to Sterilize" *OB-GYN News*, November 15, 2000.

Having invested much time and emotion in the decision process, it's easy for the sterilized person or couple to adopt a hardened stance against the Church's teaching.

Many couples drift for years before acknowledging that something between them is no longer in sync. After the initial pregnancy fear subsides, and the vision of 1001 erotic nights turns out to be something of a scam, spouse may (subtly) turn against spouse while doing their best to ignore the silent, disturbing "presence" of the choice they made. Or, worse, one spouse got sterilized without the consent of the other, which is possible under federal law protecting patient confidentiality.[17] They start to see the mystery of sexual love through the prism of stagnation. At some not-fully-conscious level, their lovemaking is no longer regarded as the great co-creative adventure God made it to be.

Archbishop Sheen called this fed-upness "black grace," the disturbing sense that God is absent, which Sheen contrasted with the white grace of God's consoling presence.[18] God is not absent, of course, but from an emotional or sensible point of view, our sinfulness impairs our capacity to experience God's consoling presence.

The Road Back Home

With the help of God's grace, however, this inner affliction can give way to a new ability to hear the still small voice of conscience. The *Catechism* teaches that "Conversion is first of all a work of the grace of God who makes our hearts return to Him: 'Restore us to thyself, O Lord, that we may

---

[17] See, for example, The Health Insurance Portability and Accountability Act (HIPAA), enacted April 14, 2003.
[18] Fulton J. Sheen, *Lift Up Your Heart* (New York: McGraw-Hill, 1950), 169–85.

be restored!'"[19] According to Christ's most famous parable, if anyone responds to the graces of repentance, the Father doesn't merely listen like a remote king: He leaps off His heavenly porch and runs to us (see Luke 15:11–32).

So repentance is not the end, but the beginning. And while it doesn't magically make the sterilization go away, there are practical options available. Although the Catholic Church, wisely, does not require sterilization reversal as a condition of God's pardon, there is an obligation to at least consider it. And many couples—in the face of long odds and financial "impossibilities," and after hearing a good priest assure them that repentance suffices—feel the Lord asking them to seek out that option.

As the beautiful stories of post-reversal babies attest, repentance can sometimes bring spectacular blessings. Few babies are cherished more deeply than post-reversal babies.[20] A wonderful organization exists to help couples financially to reverse their sterilization, called Blessed Arrows. (For more information, see Appendix.)

Whether the couple is able to have the reversal, whether they have the reversal but are unsuccessful at achieving another pregnancy—and whether or not God blesses them with another child—all of this is secondary to the momentous thing they have achieved: In one of the most delicate and profound dimensions of their lives, they have set things right with the One who made them and brought them together.

So what about men (and women) who confess the sin of sterilization, yet who truly cannot have the reversal? A unique and vexing problem arises. They may, over time, find themselves sorely tempted to delight in the very

---

[19] CCC 1432; see Lamentations 5:21.
[20] Long, *Sterilization Reversal*.

sex-without-babies mentality that led to the sterilization in the first place (otherwise known as having your cake and eating it, too).

The best pastoral advice combines common sense with mature Christian spirituality.[21] It is this: that the couple chooses to model their sex life after the same cycle of enjoyment-then-abstinence that fertile couples adopt when using NFP. This monthly time of abstinence (several days per month) is embraced as a pledge to the Lord that their rejection of the contraceptive mentality is sincere and permanent.[22] Since the tubal ligation normally does not affect menstruation, the biological signs of fertility can still be tracked as they would be in a fertile couple.

The bottom line is that deep and lasting repentance is possible after the sin of deliberate sterilization, even if no steps are taken toward a reversal. Bishop Robert Vasa of Santa Rosa, California, makes this clear: "God's infinite strength does change hearts and dispose persons to the truth who were once blind to the transcendent. Deliberate sterilization is surely a 'forgivable' sin."[23]

Seed Planting

We now address the third group of people, those who don't seem to feel the least bit guilty for having the procedure, the ones who wonder what all the fuss is about, treat the topic with levity, and make jokes about "getting snipped." Is there

---

[21] The extreme option of total abstinence is neither required by the Church nor does it enjoy a handsome track record for attracting enthusiasts.
[22] Kippley, *Sex and the Marriage Covenant*, 212–214
[23] Bishop Robert F. Vasa, JCL, "Sterilization and Full Repentance: Recovering from Intentional Contraceptive Sterilization," Appendix I in *Sterilization Reversal*.

some way to prove to them that sterilization is immoral?

Posed that way, the answer is no. As the saying goes, "only the thirsty will drink." Our approach should never be "instructive," or coming across as moralistic or superior. I would argue that it's seldom a good idea to bring it up at all, unless the other person does first. If there's an open door and you're asked for your thoughts on the matter, by all means charitably give them. Even then, instantaneous conversion is not a realistic goal.

Seed planting, however, is.

And not only seeds of truth, but also seeds of doubt as to the rightness of his or her decision. In this context, we must remember the gentleness expressed in the words of the Prophet Isaiah that began this chapter. Once people begin to realize what they've done with their gift of fertility, the full gamut of emotions can arise, including anger ("why didn't anyone tell us this before?"), grief ("I really wish I hadn't done it"), indifference ("what's done is done; whatever"), or even despair ("it's hopeless; not even God can undo the damage"). All these are human and understandable.

But regardless of subjective feelings, the Holy Spirit is always "on the air," so to speak, and He waits to be "tuned in" by those who seek Him with all their heart (Jer 29:13). May the following questions prompt new insights that the sterilized person (or the caring apologist) hasn't considered in depth:

- In my heart of hearts, did I succumb to fear or to a lack of trust in God's providence to provide for the additional children whom I believed would threaten the family's financial security?
- Is my marriage really stronger now that the "fear of pregnancy" is gone?

- Did I think deeply about our financial situation brightening, or the original circumstances that led to my sterilization vanishing?
- How much authentic Catholic teaching did we read to form our conscience? Was it just a chat with Father So-and-So, a vague "prayer for guidance," and a selective reading that favored what made us feel good about the decision? Did we bother to find out if a Church teaching even exists on the subject?
- Did anyone raise any kind of red flag of warning or caution before I went through with the decision? Did I react defensively or deny that the caution had any validity?
- Did I seriously consider the reality of bringing sterility into my next marriage if, God forbid, my spouse should die early or our marriage end some other way?
- In light of the saying of John Paul the Great that "the best gift you can give your child is a new brother or sister," has it occurred to me that, once they find out, my other children may feel robbed of younger siblings who would exist but for my decision, or even wonder deep down if he or she was really wanted?
- Have I ever looked at a baby and wondered how different things would be if I hadn't had the procedure?
- Do I have a deep and lasting peace of mind about having the vasectomy (or ligation), or do I wear a smiley face because I'm scared to face the truth, let alone bring it up with my spouse?
- Did I ever "question my questioning" about the teaching? Can I admit that I might be wrong, and two thousand years of authoritative Christian teaching might be right?

Come Lord Jesus, give me the grace to open my heart to your Holy Spirit, to surrender my life to the Father, and to live according to the plan for true happiness you have given me through your Church. Grant me humility where I have been proud, courage where I have been afraid, prudence where I have been brash, and repentance where I have been rebellious. Help me to see my fertility anew as a great gift from the Father, and to see all things in light of your Gospel. Amen

Chapter Ten

MADE, NOT BEGOTTEN
Assisted Reproductive Technologies

Our aim in this chapter is to answer why, if the Catholic Church is so pro-baby, does she then forbid the very methods that can enable infertile couples to have the babies they badly want? Have Catholics no sympathy for the pain of childless couples that are unable to conceive?

The inability to conceive can indeed be an arduous emotional and spiritual trial. Rachel's cries to her husband Jacob, "Give me children, or I shall die!" (Gen 30:1), echo in many hearts today. And these cries rightly elicit our sympathy and our support. It bears emphasizing, though, that the condition of sterility (while sometimes involving acute hardship) is not an absolute evil. Our Lord invites us to unite our sufferings to His Cross, the true source of all spiritual fecundity. Childless couples in particular, if their situation allows, "can give expression to their generosity by adopting abandoned children or performing demanding services for others" (CCC 2379).

A child is obviously a very good end, but the means to that end must also be morally good. We will explain below why some assistive reproductive technologies (ARTs)—in vitro fertilization, artificial insemination, surrogate motherhood, and cloning—are not morally good means.

Our modern view tends to see medicine—or, more grandly, Medical Science—as a panacea. In an era of rapid medical advancement, with new treatments arising for a myriad of formerly grave conditions, we have come to look at the doctor as a kind of high priest, to medical procedures as sacraments, and to the medical profession generally as a magisterium. The same people who would never dream of turning to a priest for his guidance on mononucleosis will look to a doctors for guidance on morality.

Sometimes, the medical community adopts a set of euphemisms to shade what's really going on. Language shapes attitudes, and hence perceptions. Take the difference between "reproductive" and "procreative." At first glance they seem like synonyms. Are they? To re*produce* is literally to manufacture again. It's a basically human enterprise. To procreate is a much richer concept, suggesting man's supporting role in a divine enterprise. With reproductive technology, the warm rumpled sheets of the marital bed have been replaced by crisp white smock of the lab technician. Or take "fertilized egg." This is medicalese for tiny human being, or embryo.

Another fact that has been shaded during the emotional debate surrounding ARTs is the forgotten truth is that children are a gift, not a right. The unlimited abortion license since *Roe v. Wade* has taught us to view children as disposable commodities to be welcomed, or destroyed, at will. But no one has the right to a child. If that were true, there would exist a duty somewhere to provide one.

A gift belongs in an entirely different category. Gifts can only be received, not taken. As the *Catechism* puts it, "A child is not something owed to one, but is a gift. The 'supreme gift of marriage' is a human person. A child may not be considered a piece of property, an idea to which an alleged 'right to a child' would lead. In this area, only the child possesses genuine rights: the right 'to be the fruit of the specific act of the conjugal love of his parents,' and 'the right to be respected as a person from the moment of his conception'" (2378).

The Moral Rub

As we mentioned in the Introduction, the Catholic Church has no objections to medical treatments being "artificial" per se when they assist and repair nature's flaws and diseases, e.g., eyeglasses help the eyes, hearing aids help the ears, braces help the legs, insulin helps the pancreas, and so on. Here is the rub: if a reproductive technology *assists* the marital act to achieve pregnancy, it is morally permissible. If it *replaces* it, then it is not. The latter kind of reproductive technologies do not merely compensate for nature; they commandeer it.

"Research aimed at reducing human sterility is to be encouraged," in the words of the *Catechism*, "On condition that it is placed 'at the service of the human person, of his inalienable rights, and his true and integral good according to the design and will of God'" (2375). For instance, if the woman has a blockage in her fallopian tube, "it is permitted to move the egg (through a laboratory procedure) past the blockage so that it can be fertilized through the natural marital act."[1]

Here is a sample of some kinds of ARTs that are acceptable in Catholic teaching:

---

[1] Fr. Frank Chacon and Jim Burnham, *Beginning Apologetics Vol. 5: How to Answer Tough Moral Questions: Abortion, Contraception, Euthanasia, Test-Tube Babies, Cloning and Sexual Ethics* (Farmington, NM: San Juan Catholic Seminars, 2000), 34.

- hormonal modulation of menstrual cycle irregularities;
- surgical correction of tubal damage or occlusions;
- surgical interventions to resolve endometriosis;
- use of Viagra or other male impotence medication;
- techniques designed to increases sperm count and motility;
- techniques used to resolve premature ejaculation;
- natural family planning monitoring of the signs of fertility (like cervical mucus viscosity, basal body temperature fluctuations);
- LTOT (low tubal ovum transfer), whereby eggs are retrieved and transplanted into the uterus or fallopian tube in a location favorable to fertilization; and
- NaProTechnology and its related methods of determining and restoring threats to infertility.

In vitro fertilization, donor insemination, surrogate motherhood, and cloning are all to be rejected because they violate the right of every child to be born from the fruit of a loving mother and father through the natural means of transmitting life. It is a hard saying for our society at this point, but it simply does not accord with human dignity to be the product of an impersonal biologic exchange outside the God-ordained portals of spousal love. Of course, children born through immoral means (as in the case of rape) are to be loved and cherished like any other.

Let's get into some specifics of the above ARTs.

The B-Side of *Humanae Vitae*

The main idea—or, in the parlance of the music industry, the A-side—of *Humanae Vitae* is that the natural connection between sex and babies should not be cut. In shorthand, no sex without babies. This idea, as we have seen, is a scandal to the world, a folly to dissenters, and a muddle to many since the Sixties. But there is also a B-side, which is, in a sense, even more difficult to explain to people with no appreciation of the A-side: Human beings have a right to come into existence the way God has ordained, which is through the bodily union of father and mother. It is the A-side in reverse. In shorthand, no babies without sex.

Some new reproductive technologies that have been developed in recent years, which involve highly technical medical language, but addressing them would take us far afield. (If you want to learn more about the debates over Gamete Intrafallopian Tube Transfer (GIFT), and Tubal Ovum Transfer with Sperm (TOTS), Pronuclear-stage tubal transfer (PROST), or natural cycle oocyte retrieval intravaginal fertilization (NORIF), consult the resources in the Appendix. Here we keep it as simple as possible.)

Let us begin by defining our terms. The most common form of reproductive technology is *in vitro fertilization*, or IVF. With IVF, eggs (ova) from a woman's ovary are removed and fertilized with sperm in a glass petri dish (whence the older term "test tube babies"), and then the fertilized egg (embryo, or new human being) is returned to the woman's uterus to grow until birth.[2]

---

[2] See http://www.surgeryencyclopedia.com/Fi-La/In-Vitro-Fertilization.html (accessed October 1, 2008). See also Kay Elder and Brian Dale, *In Vitro Fertilization, Second Edition* (Oxford: Cambridge University Press, 2000).

IVF (In Vitro Fertilization)

There are several grave problems with IVF. First, as we have said, the procedure opposes God's plan for the way in which children are to come into the world. A four-course dinner, a bottle of fine wine, and a candle-lit bedroom strewn with roses as a prelude to an unforgettable night of erotic communion? Not with IVF. The man masturbates into a sterilized vial, a technician mixes the sperm sample with a harvested ovum (egg) from the woman in a glass dish (*in vitro* is Latin for "in glass") in a laboratory, and then transfers the embryo, a.k.a. new human being, into the uterus. How romantic.

Second, what many people do not know is that some embryos—tiny human beings, remember—are almost always killed in the procedure. Doctors select the healthy, most "viable," embryos to implant in the womb, while the "undesirable" ones left over are either destroyed or are subject to experimentation—or they are frozen indefinitely in liquid nitrogen, consigned to what the magisterium of St. John Paul II called a perpetually "absurd fate."[3]

Third, very often more than one embryo is implanted with the hope that at least one will survive, and come to be born. Well, the majority of couples do not want twins or triplets, so when multiple siblings implant successfully, the focus of care zeroes in on the one desired baby, and the doctors will kill one or more of the others. In the womb. By abortion.

Fourth, IVF has also led to genetic engineering, "designer babies," and acceptance of the premise that "left-

---

[3] "In consequence of the fact that they have been produced *in vitro*, those embryos which art not transferred into the body of the mother and are called "spare" are exposed to an absurd fate, with no possibility of their being offered safe means of survival which can be licitly pursued." *Donum Vitae*, C.D.F, February 22, 1985, No 5.

over" embryos are fair game for experimentation. The infertile couple giveth, the infertile couple taketh away, with the help of well-paid doctors. (I haven't mentioned the cost, but it's worth noting that there is no shortage of desperate couples who spend many tens of thousands of dollars and many years of IVF dice-rolls, only to end in profound disappointment.)

Fifth, there are known health risks associated with IVF to the child (specifically twins and triplets) so conceived, including cancer, certain birth defects, and mental retardation.[4] There are no long-term studies available yet, since, as of this writing, the oldest of the more than five million people in the world conceived by IVF is 40 (Her name is Louise Brown and we'll hear more about her in a bit).

Finally, there is an even broader twofold moral problem with in vitro fertilization, and that is its close connection with the abortion industry and the attitude of the disposability of human persons it engenders. IVF involves, at the beginning, obtaining the sperm sample via masturbation; and, at the end, of harvesting many fertilized ova (again, the medicalese term for tiny babies) and picking the healthiest for implantation. The rest are discarded or frozen, exposing these tiny persons to further abuse and manipulation. It's eugenics entering the suburban form.

AI (Artificial Insemination)

The Catechism of the Catholic Church lays it out clearly. "Techniques involving only the married couple (homologous

---

[4] Medical journalist Alexandra Sifferlin summary of a giant 2013 Swedish study involving 2.5 million IVF children in the *Journal of the American Medical Association* for *Time* magazine: http://healthland.time.com/2013/07/05/how-healthy-are-ivf-babies/

artificial insemination and fertilization) are perhaps less reprehensible, yet remain morally unacceptable. They dissociate the sexual act from the procreative act. The act which brings the child into existence is no longer an act by which two persons give themselves to one another, but one that 'entrusts the life and identity of the embryo into the power of doctors and biologists and establishes the domination of technology over the origin and destiny of the human person. Such a relationship of domination is in itself contrary to the dignity and equality that must be common to parents and children'" (2377).

So there are two kinds of AI, homologous and heterologous. Homologous artificial insemination is the technique used to obtain a human conception through the transfer into the genital tracts of a married woman of the sperm previously collected from her husband. The heterologous version involves a sperm vendor (let's stop calling them donors since money typically changes hands) who is not the woman's husband. Both methods are wrong because they *replace,* or substitute, the marital act by which God has ordained as the means par excellence of transmitting human life.

With both versions, the sperm sample is collected from the man (whether married to the prospective mother or even if unknown to her) by way of masturbation and deposited into the woman's body to conceive a baby. Both IVF and DI make life without making love—the exact opposite of contraception's pattern.

Surrogate Motherhood

As the term implies, is the practice of using the womb as a rent-a-space in which a woman agrees—generally for a negotiated fee paid by a woman unable or unwilling to carry a child to term in the natural way—to bring to term a baby that belongs biologically to another couple. The disconnect between the mother-father-child unity should be obvious. For a more personally and deeply troubling angle on sperm vending, look into the work of Alana Newman, foundress of the AnonymousUs movement, made up of people who may never know their fathers, whose sperm was used in their conception (www.anonymousus.org).

Cloning

The first animal to be cloned was a tadpole, back in 1952. After Dolly the Scottish sheep (1997–2003) became a household name, a variety of larger animals have been cloned—including goats, rabbits, cows, mice, pigs, and a wild gaur—albeit with very poor results. But according to the information service of the Human Genome Project, animal cloning is expensive and notoriously ineffective. Over 90 percent of all attempts fail or lead to early death; Dolly was produced only after 276 failed attempts.[5]

While *human cloning* has not yet been successfully done, at least not brought to birth, maverick scientists are slouching toward that goal line.[6] Cloning involves produc-

---

[5] Human Genome Program, "Human Genome Project Information," US Department of Energy, http://www.ornl.gov/sci/techresources/Human_Genome/elsi/cloning.shtml.

[6] Samuel H. Wood, CEO of Stemagen in La Jolla, CA, claimed in January, 2008, to have manufactured five cloned embryos from his own skin cells. These were destroyed before implantation. See http://www.washingtonpost.com/wp-dyn/content/article/2008/01/17/AR2008011700324.html?hpid=topnews. For a succinct treatment of how Christian moral principles are applied to these technologies, see Janet E. Smith and Christopher Kaczor, *Life Issues, Medical Choices: Questions and Answers For Catholics* (Cincinnati: Servant Books, 2007), pp. 60-73; and Marie Anderson, M.D., FACOG and John Bruchalski, M.D., *Assisted Reproductive Technologies are Anti-*

ing a new living being by inserting the genetic material from the nucleus of a donor parent cell into an egg that has had its nucleus removed. When that dual combination is stimulated electrically or chemically, the result is an identical twin of the original donor. Theoretically, there is no limit to the number of cloned organisms drawn from the genetic information of the adult donor. So far, the unfettered capitalists have not yet found a profit motive to justify going full-tilt with cloning technology. Give them time. They are not missionaries but mercenaries.

Are You My Mother?

Millions of children have enjoyed P. D. Eastman's storybook, *Are You My Mother?* It's about a little bird that has been separated from his mother and wanders the landscape trying to discover his own, and his mother's, true identity. The story is an unintended metaphor for the havoc wreaked upon children and their putative parents by reproductive technologies. When lab technicians, doctors, paid surrogates, and other parties outside the mother and the father get involved in bringing a child into the world, the forgotten person is the child. Also disregarded is what coming-to-be from multiple "parents" and "techniques" does to his or her sense of identity. Scant research has been done in this area.

What the above technologies have in common is the same unnatural separation between sex and babies that is condemned by *Humanae Vitae*. They each seek the kite of life without the string of love, the rose's scent without the rose, the music without the melody. And whether considered

---

Woman, available online at http://www.usccb.org/prolife/programs/rlp/04anderson.shtml.

singly or together (they often overlap in practice) these technologies invariably lead to troublesome legal quagmires. The courts are becoming clogged with examples. Here are four:

First, Janet Smith documents a case in which a woman got herself pregnant through DI using her husband's frozen sperm, and they later divorced. The woman sued him for child support, but his attorneys won the day when the court determined that the legal father was not the ex-husband but the lab technician who had performed the insemination procedure, an act, said the judge, that was the proximate cause of her becoming pregnant.[7]

Second, in a television interview, the late ex-abortionist (and Catholic convert) Dr. Bernard Nathanson related a story to Fr. Frank Pavone of Priests For Life regarding a California trial that sounds more like a Monty Python sketch than a real life case. An infertile couple (where both partners were sterile) hired a reproductive technologist to mix a male donor's sperm with a female donor's egg. The resultant embryo was implanted in the womb of yet another party (a surrogate mother) and she delivered the baby nine months later. Still follow? At the time of the trial, the child was eight. The litigation was meant to answer the legal question, "Who are the parents?" As that question began to be asked, the original couple that paid for all this . . . filed for divorce. Who indeed are the parents? The original adoptive couple? The sperm donor and the egg benefactress? The implantee? Legally speaking, it's a moot question. The judge eventually placed the child in a foster home.[8]

---

[7] See Janet Smith, "Reproductive Technologies," in *Encyclopedia of Catholic Doctrine* ed. by Russell Shaw (Huntington, IN: Our Sunday Visitor, 1997), 576-579.

[8] For the entire transcript, see http://www.priestsforlife.org/testimony/nathanson.html.

Third, a heartrending trial in Vermont showed how the insinuation of reproductive technologies into already difficult conflicts aggravates them and multiplies their evil effects. In 2008, a Vermont judge declared that the ex-lesbian partner is the rightful mother to another woman's biological six-year-old daughter. The biological mother, Lisa Miller, became an evangelical Christian and left the lesbian lifestyle when the baby, Isabella, was seventeen months old. Janet Jenkins, Miller's female lover at the time, sought full custody of the baby, claiming she was a parent even though she was not biologically related to Isabella and had not sought to adopt her.

A Vermont judge declared that Isabella has two mommies; and appellate courts in Virginia (the state where Isabella was born and has lived most of her life) directed Virginia to fully recognize the Vermont orders giving the ex-lesbian partner (Vermont resident Janet Jenkins) wide unsupervised visitation rights. How was Isabella conceived? By in vitro fertilization when Miller and Jenkins were in a civil union over six years before. On November 20, 2009, a judge found Miller in contempt of court for continuing to deny Jenkins access to her daughter, then seven years old. Authorities ordered Lisa Miller to give her daughter Isabella to Janet Jenkins on New Year's Day, 2010. Miller refused and, as of this writing, remains a fugitive with the little girl.[9]

Finally, as of this writing, a girl in New York is stuck in the foster care system despite the fact that her biological father is a fit parent who desires access and care for her. But the court does not recognize him as her father. The girl has

---

[9] Erick Eckholm, "New Charges in Virginia Kidnapping Over Custody, *The New York Times,* Oct. 8, 2014. https://www.nytimes.com/2014/10/09/us/new-charges-are-brought-in-same-sex-custody-case.html.

remained in foster care since 2015 because her mother is in a lesbian relationship with neglect petitions pending against both the mother and her lover. The five-judge panel do not deny that the girl's foster care status was "relevant" and "concerning," but they still denied the father's request to prove his fatherhood. He donated his sperm as a kind of humanitarian gesture and now wants to make things right. But he's not a father in any relevant sense because . . . the court says so.[10]

These pretzel-like visions of chaos show how reproductive technologies strike at the very foundation of marriage, of family and parenthood. Further, at stake are not merely arcane legal disputes but the very idea of personhood. The question "Who am I?" is closely tied to others such as, "Whose son am I?" "Who is my father?" "How did I come to be?" The end game in all this is total chaos over how, and with whom, we ought to pass on human life.

The sheer ability to medically intervene doesn't necessarily justify intervention. All science comes with ethical limits, as Aldous Huxley's *Brave New World*, Mary Shelley's *Frankenstein*, and the prescient 1997 movie *Gattaca*, remind us. Examples of the truism could be multiplied.

The reproductive technologies under discussion represent a relatively new challenge for the teaching Church, spawned as they were in the same era that produced the bloodiest wars, the shadow of nuclear annihilation, the unlimited abortion license, hardcore pornography, no-fault divorce, and the rise of a new global persecution of believers unmatched perhaps since Roman times.

---

[10] Dr. Jennifer Roback-Morse, "New York Court: A Girl's Right to Her Father Doesn't Matter: Protecting 'Marriage Equality' Does," in *The Stream*, February 9, 2018. URL: https://stream.org/child-child-government-says/.

The Three *Vitaes*

Each era of Church history, brings new challenges to the Church as Teacher. You can chart how this has played out in the last fifty years as time has gone from march to mad dash:

- The sexual revolution exploded and the world became preoccupied with the new borderless sexual appetite. In 1968, against vehement opposition even within the Church, Pope Paul VI wrote *Humanae Vitae* as a bulwark against the rising tide of confusion and promiscuity.
- As new reproductive technologies appeared in the 1970s and 80s, a new obsession with pursuing parenthood while bypassing God's plan for sexuality. In 1987, the Congregation for the Doctrine of the Faith issued the important, if lesser known, document titled *Instruction on Respect for Human Life in Its Origin and on the Dignity of Procreation*
- *Donum Vitae* ("the gift of life"), which sets forth the moral principles for evaluating these procedures in light of natural law and the constant teaching of the Church, and was signed by the Prefect of the CDF, Joseph Cardinal Ratzinger, now Pope Emeritus Benedict XVI.
- As time rolled on, as a new penchant for killing frail, vulnerable human beings took hold in the form of abortion on demand right up until the moment of birth, St. John Paul the Great published *Evangelium Vitae* ("the Gospel of Life") in response to the world's new penchant for killing human beings.

These three successive attacks—upon marriage and the beauty of human sexuality, upon the right of the child to be born from the love-union of his parents, and finally the attack upon human life itself—were answered by the Church in her defense of the rights of the marriage bed, the rights of children, and the very right to life, respectively. Serious Christians are called to embrace this answer and make it their own.[11] We await from the magisterium the next round of doctrinal fortifications regarding transgender ideology, the redefinition of marriage, and the push toward human cloning.

The *Catechism* quotes generously from all three "*Vitaes*" in its sections on marriage. "Techniques that entail the dissociation of husband and wife, by the intrusion of a person other than the couple (donation of sperm or ovum, surrogate uterus), are gravely immoral. These techniques (heterologous artificial insemination and fertilization) infringe upon the child's right to be born of a father and mother known to him and bound to each other by marriage. They betray the spouses' 'right to become a father and a mother only through each other'" (2376).

The 1860s error of the Victorians said that the ickiness of sex could only be redeemed by the intention of a baby. A hundred years later, the 1960s error of the Hedonists shouted from the rooftops that sex and babies have no inherent connection at all, and have divorced amicably, thank you! As we said in Chapter One, this separation of sex from babies

---

[11] I am indebted here to Msgr. Philip J. Reilly for his insights into the meaning of the three *Vitaes* during a 2006 talk given in Fatima, Portugal, titled "*Humanae Vitae* and *Donum Vitae*." Additionally, on September 8, 2008, the Congregation for the Doctrine of the Faith released an important Instruction titled *Dignitas Personae*, found here: http://www.vatican.va/roman_curia/congregations/cfaith/documents/rc_con_cfaith_doc_20081208_dignitas-personae_en.html.

led directly to the "ideal" of "free" "love" and the cult of the non-procreative orgasm.

By one of those "God-incidences," on July 25, 1978, Pope Paul VI was vindicated ten years to the day after *Humanae Vitae* debuted. That day, twelve days before the Pontiff died, Louise Brown of England was born—the world's first IVF baby. You can draw a straight short line from Louise Brown to "octomom" Nadya Shuleman. (Remember her?) Leave it to a culture of death to think it can produce life without God. A hyper-sexualized, pornified, anti-baby culture that now excels at inventing technologies that make babies without sex? Irony.

A brave new world will continue to carve itself out if we ignore the historic Christian vision of human sexuality in all its integrity, beauty, and order. The micro is the macro. The person shapes the couple, the couple shapes the family; and the family, for good or for ill, shapes the society.

Art sometimes succeeds where arguments fail. Stevie Wonder's 1975 hit song "Isn't She Lovely" is a tribute to his newborn daughter. In it, he articulates beautifully, if inadvertently, the Catholic intuition of the unity between love and life and of the exquisite splendor of the truth:

> *I can't believe what God has done*
> *Through us he's given life to one*
> *But isn't she lovely, made from love*

Chapter Eleven

N.F.P. VS. A.B.C.
The Moral Differences between Natural Family Planning and Artificial Birth Control

In rejecting contraception while yet condoning natural family planning, the Catholic Church has been accused of either playing a silly word game, or of making a distinction without a difference. After all, in both cases a couple combines the same two realities: an active sex life and the avoidance of becoming pregnant. How can the first case be wrong and the second right?

The difference lies in the means. The ends (no matter how good) neither justify the means nor homogenize them. We find examples of this all the time in everyday life. One couple wants to buy a summer cottage, so they work hard and save, until they finally have enough cash to buy one. Another couple also wants a cottage but they sell drugs. Same ends, different means. Or, one student wants an A+, so he studies long hours and hires a tutor. Another cheats and plagiarizes. Same ends, different means.

Contraception is the introduction of a note of separation

and alienation into the heart of what is supposed to be an act of supreme intimacy and oneness. Its message is, "The two shall *not* be one." And its main business is that of thwarting, preventing, undermining, blocking, sabotaging, hindering, foiling, inhibiting, and defeating an act exchange that, by its nature, is ordered to a great good: the coming to be of a new human person.

Against vs. For

Notice the similarity between the word "contradict," which literally means "against the speaking," and the word "contraception," which, as we saw in the introduction, means "against the beginning." Objectively speaking, contraception is the repudiation of the adventure of parenthood. By raising up a two-sided mirror between the spouses, contraception is a gussied-up form of mutual masturbation.

The couple knows deep down that a baby could result from a contracepted act of intercourse. They would not necessarily choose abortion; indeed, they may even shrink in horror at the thought. A baby who "slips through" the phalanx of birth control security guards and is born, however, is by definition an unwanted baby—even if he or she is later kept and loved. How so? Because the very existence of the baby was considered and rejected through the decision to disable their sex act so that it would *not* do what it's supposed to do.

How does all this compare with NFP?

It must be admitted that it's possible for a couple to misuse natural family planning by declining to view their fertility as a gift and thus to adopt an outlook similar to the contraceptive mentality. Say, for example, a couple with no known sterility problems is married for ten years. They have a heated pool, a big house, three cars, an annual Costa Rica vacation, and yet they endlessly postpone children with no serious reason. That couple would clearly not be acting in harmony with the message of *Humanae Vitae*. Still, they sin more by omission than by commission. They may be stingy or fearful of their fertility, but this is different altogether from the sin of contraception.

St. Pope John Paul II zeroed in on the difference between birth prevention and birth regulation in his apostolic exhortation on the Christian family, *Familiaris Consortio* (1981). The following passage is a good example of what happens when you think deeply, and not just feel deeply, about the important things in life. The Holy Father approaches the issue by asking how it affects the persons involved from a subjective perspective, which is quite different than from an objective law or doctrine perspective. Characteristically dense but rich in meaning, he is worth quoting at some length:

> When couples, by means of recourse to contraception, separate these two meanings that God the Creator has inscribed in the being of man and woman and in the dynamism of their sexual communion, they act as "arbiters" of the divine plan and they "manipulate" and degrade human sexuality—and with it themselves and their married partner—by altering its value of "total" self-giving. Thus the innate language that expresses the total reciprocal self-giving of husband and wife is overlaid, through contraception, by an objectively contradictory language, namely, that of not giving oneself totally to the other. This leads not only to a positive refusal to be open to life but also to a falsification of the inner truth of conjugal love, which is called upon to give itself in personal totality.

> When, instead, by means of recourse to periods of infertility, the couple respect the inseparable connection between the unitive and procreative meanings of human sexuality, they are acting as "ministers" of God's plan and they "benefit from" their sexuality according to the original dynamism of "total" self-giving, without manipulation or alteration. (FC 32)

Notice the contrast the Holy Father makes here between the contracepting couple being *arbiters* who *manipulate*, and couples using NFP who are *ministers* of God's plan who experience the *total self-giving* through respecting both meanings of sex. The contrast shows an oil-and-water difference both in subjective attitude and in objective behavior. He then concludes:

> In the light of the experience of many couples and of the data provided by the different human sciences, theological reflection is able to perceive and is called to study further the difference, both anthropological and moral, between contraception and recourse to the rhythm of the cycle: it is a difference which is much wider and states that the two mentalities at work in the two means of birth regulation reflect two entirely different anthropologies. (FC 32)

Unwanted vs. Unplanned

During discussions about birth control and NFP, you might hear it said, "The Church teaches you have to have grave reasons to avoid pregnancy." This or similar phrasings imply that the standard to justify recourse to NFP is very high, as though you have to have blood coming out your ears or have some incapacitating mental or physical illness, or possibly alien abduction.

This is untrue. The problem lies with the first English translation published for a wide English-speaking audience by the Daughters of St. Paul. Where the text, speaking to reasons and motives, has *iustae rationes* (HV 10) and *iustae causae* (HV 16), the word grave was used. This is made slightly more complicated by the fact that the Italian translation has *gravi*, which seems to suggest grave in English. The more rigorist folks who insist on "grave reasons" point out that Pope Pius XII used *gravi* in his 1951 speech to Italian midwives. He did, but his remarks a) were not addressed to the universal Church and have to be seen in the context of the Pope's mother tongue, Italian, and b) Latin is the official language of the Church. Then Cardinal Wojtyla, later John Paul II, wrote an essay in 1969 in which he drops "grave motives" and uses "serious causes" from the Latin.[1]

The correct sense of this is to say the couple must have just, or sufficiently serious (i.e., not for frivolous or materialistic) reasons to have recourse to NFP. While the Church wisely does not lay down explicit dos and don'ts, nor provide a specific criteria list, Paul VI alludes to reasons "based on the physical or psychological condition of the spouses or on external factors" (HV 16).

If NFP couples have such reasons to avoid bringing a new child into the world at a given time, they simply monitor the bodily signs of female fertility, and, during days known to be

---

[1] Karol Cardinal Wojtyla, "Crisis in Morality." *Crisis in Morality: The Vatican Speaks Out.* (Washington, DC: United States Catholic Conference, 1969) p. 4., quoted by Angela Dr. Bonilla in "*Humanae Vitae*: Grave Motives To Use a Good Translation" in *Homiletic and Pastoral Review*, March 25, 2008. URL: http://www.hprweb.com/2008/03/humanae-vitae-grave-motives-to-use-a-good-translation/.

fertile, they choose to show their love in non-genital ways. (Short list of suggestions: play backgammon, take a beach walk, go bowling, read your favorite respective books by a crackling fire together, pray the Rosary, watch a Frank Capra movie, learn photography.) Then, each and every time they bodily renew their marriage covenant, they are open to new life, even if they foreknow that chances are slim that they will conceive during sex in the infertile period. Using a poker comparison, such couples treat God as a partner with whom they're willing to share high-value cards, whereas contracepting couples treat God as an opponent they want to defeat. Another way to say this is to say that NFP couples never have unwanted children, only sometimes unplanned ones.

Some claim that sex on a day known to be infertile is the same thing as using birth control in general. The key difference is that God Himself designed the human female with a natural rhythm of fertility and infertility, and this knowledge merely determines the timing of an act of intercourse. It doesn't involve the desecration of any such acts.

God arranged this monthly ebb and flow. His creatures are free to enter into its dance, either genitally or non-genitally as their life situation warrants. Most people don't look at it this way, but since ovulation occurs only one day a month (abstention usually lasts five to ten days, depending on the duration of the fertile phase), the divine design actually favors the enjoyment of unity and sexual satisfaction over the procreative meaning by a hefty margin!

The attack on the unitive meaning is also real, but it's subtle and more difficult to prove. This does not make it less real. If you sit in the same room with an exposed chunk of radium, you're really being affected by the radiation even though you may feel absolutely no sensible reaction. An invisible effect is not the same as a non-existent one.

The exact opposite of this would be the Real Presence of Jesus in the Eucharist. Even though a battery of biochemical tests done to the consecrated Host would detect nothing beyond the accidental qualities of unleavened bread, Jesus taught us He is really *there*, and that the species of bread are really *not there*.

In the use of NFP, not one sex act is ever manipulated or thwarted. What such couples say to God is, "Father, we have prayerfully discerned our life situation and we believe we ought not conceive at this time. But we want to honor you as the true Lord of Life. In partnership with you, we enter into this embrace trusting that, if it be your will to bless it with a child, we will joyfully accept him or her." On fertile days, they do stuff not involving the genitals. Start that list with Scrabble.

NFP involves the pursuit of goods other than the good of a new human being. Contraception involves sterilizing an act of intercourse that is feared to be fertile. Beyond noting the biological signs of fertility, NFP involves no action at all. In this case, a non-action is not immoral. NFP is non-procreative sex; contraception is anti-procreative sex.

If the Catholic Church really taught that couples must consciously wish that each and every act of intercourse result in pregnancy, then the doctrine would forbid intercourse on infertile days!

Hidden Benefits Galore

There is solid statistical evidence that couples living the NFP lifestyle are far, far less likely to divorce than those using birth control. Elzbieta Wojcik cites the extraordinary finding by an Austrian doctor named Josef Rotzer who tracked fourteen hundred NFP users over twenty years and found a divorce rate among them of *zero percent*.² There has not yet been a large amount of objective research done on the role of birth control in the skyrocketing divorce rate since the late 1960s, although sociologist Robert Michael attributes roughly half of all divorces to the explosion of contraceptive use in the decade that straddled *Humanae Vitae*.³

It takes a certain combination of blindness and boldness to refuse to see the causal role played by contraception in the high divorce rate, which sprouted up after *Humanae Vitae* was thrown under the bus. The Holy Father himself saw it coming:

> Indeed it is to be feared that husbands who become accustomed to contraceptive practices will lose respect for their wives. They may come to disregard their wives' psychological and physical equilibrium and use their wives as instruments for serving their own desires. (HV 17)

How vindicated he has been as a prophet. Surveying the emotional and social wreckage fifty years later, we can see that the causal connection is not so mysterious or impossible to discern. Ironically, much of the research documenting the empirical evidence for a causal connection to social disruptions and marital strains over the past fifty years has been done by secular scientists.⁴ If the only reason for marital

---

[2] Elzbieta Wojcik, "Natural Regulation of Conception and Contraception," *International Review of Natural Family Planning* 9:4, cited in Smith, *Humanae Vitae*, 390. See also Nona Aquilar, *The New No-Pill, No Risk Birth Control* (New York: Rawson Associates, 1986), 186–191.
[3] Ibid., 391.
[4] For an extended review of this evidence, see Mary Eberstadt, "The Vindication of *Humanae Vitae*" in *First Things*, August/September, 2008, http://www.firstthings.com/article.php3?id_article=6262.

stability is that most are serious Catholics who accept the teaching of Jesus on the indissolubility of marriage, why do other "serious Catholics," who yet dissent from *Humanae Vitae*, divorce at higher rates than their NFP-loving Catholic brethren?

The answer is, there is something more profound at work here. Couples who use NFP must have an all-important conversation each month. Will we have another baby? Why not? They regularly tap into the very reality that differentiates their relationship from every other relationship. The natural cycle of the wife, with its silent rhythm of *now* and *not yet*, becomes the object of intimate and even affectionate knowledge of the couple. When they renew their marriage in sexual union, they are free from worrying about whether their effort to sabotage it will fail. With *sex au naturel*— which involves the refusal to throw pills and chemicals at communication problems—this mental intrusion does not exist. They're *open*.

On the other hand, contracepting couples have no heightened expectation of pregnancy during fertile days, and hence no monthly conversation about new babies. Their sex life—which was supposed to ignite into erotic delights only dreamed of by Viagra ad men—can easily peter out over time. If unbridled, always available sexual experience made people happy, we would be the happiest society in human history.

By contrast, NFP couples tend to be allergic to the very language of birth control, which is to say, the language of protection. Think about what this communicates. Protection implies some harm from which we want to protect against. In the winter, we need protection against the cold; in summer, against the heat; in war, against the enemy. Sexual intercourse, says birth control, needs protection from the potential alien invader otherwise known as Junior.

Contraception has not-so-subtly redefined children as the unspoken enemy of true romance.

Analogies "R" Us

We close with five simple analogies that highlight the moral difference between natural family planning and contraception:

Dieting. I don't know the origin of this one, and, like all analogies, it's not perfect, but it makes instant sense to most people when they hear it. We touched on it in Chapter Six. Eating is to the individual what sexual intercourse is to the race: each sustains. But if you want to lose weight, you diet (i.e., you abstain from food). You don't eat and then stick a spoon down your throat to induce vomiting. Such a person acts in a way that appears to respect the natural end of eating, but then frustrates its power while simultaneously enjoying its pleasure. This condition is called bulimia, which is an eating disorder. In light of natural law, contraception is a sexual disorder.

Speaking. Mary Rosera Joyce develops this at some length, in one of the earliest philosophical defenses of *Humanae Vitae*.[5] We all recognize that others deserve to hear the truth from us when we speak to them, especially our close friends and family. But some occasions call for silence or prudence, as when a technically "truthful" word would hurt the person. Still, we must never lie, which is the use of words to deceive another. Silence is not the same as lying.

In this analogy, contraception is the equivalent of lying; NFP the equivalent of remaining silent. John Paul II sums

---

[5] Mary Rosera Joyce, *The Meaning of Contraception* (New York: Alba House, 1970), 41.

this up by saying that the body has its own language of love, and contraception is its lie.

Praying. The first principle in any spiritual life is that one must pray. Prayer is the lifeblood of one's relationship with God, calling out to Him by name, mentally affirming one's love for Him. But at times in daily life (the majority of the time, actually), we cannot pray directly or consciously. Yet we must never fake it for show. Obviously, we must not blaspheme, either by taking the Lord's name in vain or by playacting. On the bodily, interpersonal level, contraception is a kind of blasphemy.

Protesting. The late English philosopher G.E.M. Anscombe, mentioned in Chapter Two, painted a picture of disgruntled factory workers who have legitimate complaints against management.[6] They can choose two ways of expressing them. They can implement a work-to-rule strategy and resolve to work at a minimal speed, which would slow down production, bring profits down, and force management to cough up some justice. Or they can wander through the factory destroying equipment as a way of expressing their gripe. Same message; different means. The former workers are like NFP (a legitimate end is achieved through non-action), the latter like contraception (the same end achieved through an additional anti-life act).

Wedding Planning. Professor Donald DeMarco asks us to imagine two pairs of engaged couples who are planning their wedding reception. In both cases, the hall is too small to hold all their friends, so they must pick a limited number of attendees. Couple A mails invitation cards to their chosen friends. (They'd like the others to be there but the space limitation forbids it.) Couple B also sends out cards to those

---

[6] Anscombe, *Contraception and Chastity*, 20.

whom they invite, but then they also mail other cards to the people whom they couldn't invite, which read, "Please do not come to our wedding reception."

Couple A acts with an NFP mindset in which non-attendees don't receive the "stay away" cards. Couple B acts with a contraceptive mindset in which the non-invitation is joined by an action designed to make extra sure they aren't there. In the analogy, God is the friend who is positively excluded from being present, so to speak, to bless the act of intercourse.

I give the last word to Venerable Fulton J. Sheen:

> Is my eye finding the best self-expression when it is blindfolded? Is my ear delighted in its individuality when it is plugged? Is my tongue finding its noblest expression when my mouth is bandaged? When then should I say that husband and wife are finding their individuality and best expressing themselves when they stifle, frustrate, and contracept those faculties which God has given to them, and through which they may find an expression so genuine that their own individuality stands incarnate before them? The deepest wound one could have inflicted upon Michelangelo or Raphael would have been to tell either of them that a certain work of his did not measure up to the possibilities of his genius; so, too, a husband and wife who have the slightest pride in the creative artistry of their lives should deem their lives a failure if they have fallen short of what might have been expected of them, and certainly nothing can be more reasonably expected of life than life.[7]

---

[7] Fulton J. Sheen, *Old Errors and New Labels* (New York: Alba House, 2007), 184–85.

EPILOGUE

After speaking at a conference in the Midwest, I was at the product table signing books and answering questions from the attendees that milled about. A quiet couple in their early-thirties lingered near the fringes of the crowd; the mother was gently bouncing a baby in her arms. As the crowd thinned and I was getting ready to leave, they came over and introduced themselves. "Your book changed our marriage and our lives," the dad told me.

"Now that's music to an author's ears," I replied, and I asked them what it was about the book that touched them. They looked at each other and broke into identical grins. "We were married for ten years and were totally on board with contraception," the mother explained. "We hadn't heard otherwise from anywhere in the Church and when my husband and I saw you talk about your escape from the ideology of dissent with Marcus Grodi on EWTN's *The Journey Home*, we realized God was calling us to make a change. So we did. And our baby boy, Cy, here is the result."

There are no words to describe the experience of meeting little Cy, getting my picture taken with the little man and his new mom and dad. I still have the photo.

It's easy to focus on argumentation, theory, theology, and other seemingly abstract things when discussing contraception. But since it impinges upon the very foundation of every human life, there is an intensely personal, historical side to the discussion. That young couple's family tree is changed forever because Cy is now with them. And that is so because they heard the message that love and life belong together and that God always sends a loaf of bread down with each baby. Cy may even have a new brother or sister by now for all I know. Whole worlds come into being—or fail to do so—based on the decision to say yes or no to the life-stifling nature of contraception.

The teaching of *Humanae Vitae* spills over into other areas or life beyond the experience of couples. The teaching of *Humanae Vitae* is one of the few true litmus tests for orthodoxy. If you accept it, you are virtually sure to accept everything else the Church teaches about sex, from homosexuality to the redefinition of marriage to fornication, masturbation, and the impossibility of female priests. If you reject it, you are virtually sure to "have a problem with it" (weaselly code for "I think its hooey but I want to appear faithful."[1]

I'm sorry, but there are no half-measures. The teaching is true or it is false. If it is true, I must conform myself to its norms; if it is false, the Catholicism is worse than a false religion—it is diabolically evil. (*What?* Bind the consciences of billions of people for two-thousand years over something so intimate and personal, and *get it wrong*?)

---

[1] A sad little book peddles this idea, titled "*Why You Can Disagree and Remain a Faithful Catholic*" by the late bow-tie sporting Benedictine monk named Philip Kaufman, featuring a Foreword by the dissenter Robert McCormick, SJ, whom I mentioned in Chapter One.

EPILOGUE

For me, it was the incisive, contrarian nature of the thing—its bold willingness to be a fool for Christ in the middle of an army of hedonists—that drew me to its bracing message. Christians are supposed to stand out in a certain way, are called to be a peculiar people. Well, brother, saying no to birth control and yes to both birth and (self) control, will certainly make you stand out as peculiar in a world of Kardashians.

And this rings biblically true, too, incorporating as it does both Covenants. The elegant King James Version tells it, "For thou art an holy people unto the Lord thy God, and the Lord hath chosen thee to be a *peculiar people* unto Himself, above all the nations that *are* upon the earth" (Deut 14:2). The first pope reinforced this calling for the New Israel, the Church: "But ye are a chosen generation, a royal priesthood, an holy nation, a *peculiar people*; that ye should shew forth the praises of Him who hath called you out of darkness into his marvelous light" (1 Pet 2:9).

There is a lot of compromising going in the Christian world. I'm not saying Catholics are immune from the compromising game, but there is a difference is: the teachings of the Church cannot change because they come from Christ. This bedrock certainty is not found (despite so much sacramental and liturgical unity) in Eastern Orthodoxy, nor in any form of Protestantism, but only in the Catholic Church, where what Christ intends for humanity—including the full truth about sex and marriage—is preserved and protected, irrespective of what a majority may opine or even what some Synod fathers may assert. Not teaching clearly on a particular doctrine does not imply the doctrine is false. Venerable Fulton J. Sheen got this exactly right when he announced on his hugely popular TV show in 1953, "Moral principles do not depend on a majority vote. Wrong is wrong, even if everybody is wrong. Right is right, even if nobody is right."[2]

This is in the objective order, of course. In the subjective, we must always bear in mind that most people today (especially under the age of thirty) have become so inured to sexual violence, so over-exposed to the ubiquity of pornography, and so tangled in the emotional fallout from the no-fault divorce culture that they deeply want to be understood before they'll hear any preaching about objective morality.

There are a lot of "bruised reeds and smoldering wicks" (Isa 42:3) walking around college campuses and in workplaces today. Sexual woundedness is pandemic. The maxim attributed to Plato fits snugly here: "Be kind to everyone you meet because everyone you meet is fighting a great battle." Kindness has a kind of magic in it. It disarms the defensive and the angry. "A soft answer," says the Proverb, "turns away wrath" (15:1).

To briefly review, the thesis of this book is that the rejection of two millennia of Christian teaching on a sphere of human life that goes to the marrow of the emotional and bodily life has opened up not just one box with the name Pandora on the side, but a whole set of Russian Matryoshka dolls, each exposing a new sphere of disruptive consequences: "no-fault" (is there a crazier oxymoron?) divorce and the lifelong suffering of the children of divorce,[3] the scourge of abortion, the normalization of homosexual behavior, the rise of hardcore porn (with its the jet-fuel delivery system: the Internet), the redefinition of marriage, forced speech regarding the new "non-binary" pronouns

---

[2] Fulton J. Sheen, *Life Is Worth Living* television broadcast, Program 19.
[3] See Leila Miller, *Primal Loss: The Now-Adult Children of Divorce Speak* (LCB Publishing: Phoenix), 2017, and my interview with her: https://www.patrickcoffin.media/my-parents-divorce-hurts/

EPILOGUE

(ze, hir, sie, they, etc.), the astoundingly successful spread of transgender ideology through the mass media, the #metoo movement with its seemingly endless line up of male predators in Hollywood. (I have wondered why it wasn't called the #himtoo movement so as to focus on the perpetrator rather than the victim.)

Ultimately, all dissent from the norms of *Humanae Vitae* comes down to the spirit of divorce, of splitting and sundering. In contraception, as we have seen, love is split from life. But this split did not arise in isolation. In the first thousand years of Christianity, there was unity, then the East-West schism happened and the papacy (a fundamental father figure) was rejected.

Roughly speaking, five hundred years later, the so-called Reformation happened and Christ was split from the Church and the latter was rejected.

The splitting continued. Two hundred-fifty years later, the Enlightenment happened and reason was divorced from faith and the latter was rejected.

These unnatural separations set the pattern for the future ones: love from life in the Lambeth Conference decision to allow Anglicans to contracept; husband from wife in literal divorce; mother from child in Roe v. Wade; male from female in homosexuality; and now the split within the very Self in transgenderism.

The Gospel message is the efficacious antidote to all disunity. It is the norm of restoration and unity. How can we reach people with the fullness of that Gospel without turning people off with by "rules" and "dogmas," however true they may be?

What if we started with the very longing inherent in sexual desire?

As we said in the Introduction, evil is not a substance. People who commit sexual sin are looking for *something*. They're chasing down their desires, fallen as they are, to find what they're looking for, to achieve some kind of satisfaction or fulfillment.

Of course, apart from God's plan, their strategy will ultimately fail. But if we begin the conversation with that longing, that misdirected yearning that ends up missing the mark, and talk about what it might imply for the reason why we exist at all.[4] There is a saying that is (falsely) attributed to G. K. Chesterton, which gets at this notion: "A man knocking on the door of a brothel is looking for God."[5] The fact that we keep falling for the false substitutes doesn't mean the Real Thing doesn't exist.

Author and professor of government J. Budzisewski eloquently describes how this heart-pangy longing relates not so much to our search for God but His for us:

> We severed rings do not have the power to reattach ourselves to the magnet. The magnet must reattach to us. When at last each atom and each grain have rotated to face the Suffering God, ring after ring in order, the severed parts of our own hearts reunite; and as Man is reunited with himself, so he is reunited with his other self, who is Woman.[6]

---

[4] The New Testament Greek word for sin, *hamartia*, means to miss the mark.
[5] The actual source, or closely resembling it, is *The World, the Flesh, and Father Smith* by Bruce Marshall (Houghton Mifflin: 1945), p. 108, cited in *The American Chesterton Society*, URL: https://www.chesterton.org/other-quotations/
[6] J. Budziszewski, *On the Meaning of Sex* (Wilmington: ISI Books) 2012, p. 143–44.

EPILOGUE

Each perishable beauty serves as a signpost pointing up and away to a Beauty that does not perish. The key that unlocks the riches of the ancient Christian sexual ethic is this: by obeying its norms we are led not into servile frustration but into that rapturous union with the divine Bridegroom who wooed us first and won us on the cross. Then, when the sacramental two-in-one-flesh bond on earth has ended, we shall know as we are known and see as we are seen by the Author of all love (1 Cor 13:12). Which is why heaven is called the Beatific Vision.

APPENDIX

Natural Family Planning

Billings Ovulation Method:

- *The Billings Method: Controlling Fertility without Drugs or Devices*, by Evelyn Billings, MD, and Ann Westmore
www.boma-usa.org
- *Family of the Americas Foundation*
P.O. Box 1170
Dunkirk, MD 20754
(301) 627-3346
www.familyplanning.net
familyplanning@yahoo.com

Creighton Model:

- For resources and links to the work of Dr. Thomas Hilgers, MD, co-developer of the Creighton Model and specialist in female infertility:
Pope Paul Institute for the Study of Human Reproduction
6901 Mercy Rd.
Omaha, NE 68106
(402) 390-6600
www.creightonmodel.com

www.popepaulvi.com
www.naprotechnology.com

Sympto-Thermal Method:

- *The Art of Natural Family Planning*, by John and Sheila Kippley
  The Couple to Couple League International
  P.O. Box 111184
  Cincinnati, OH 45211-1184
  www.ccli.org
- *Serena*, a Canadian organization that teaches the SymptoThermal Method
  www.serena.ca

Theology of the Body

- *Theology of the Body for Beginners*, by Christopher West. See also www.theologyofthebody.com.
- *Theology of the Body Made Simple*, by Anthony Percy and Kenneth Schmitz
- *Men and Women Are from Eden: A Study Guide to John Paul II's Theology of the Body*, by Dr. Mary Healy
- *Male and Female He Created Them: A Theology of the Body*, original writings of Karol Wojtyla translated by Dr. Michael Waldstein (with commentary)
- *Theology of the Body: What It Means, Why It Matters*, by Fr. Richard M. Hogan
- *Freedom: Twelve Lives Transformed by the Theology of the Body*, ed. by Matthew Pinto, Foreword by Christopher West

APPENDIX

Catholic Teaching on Sex and Marriage

- *Through Sex to Love: Escape From the Emotional Wasteland of Recreational Sex,* by John H. McGoey, SFM
- *Collapse of the Sexual Revolution: The Remedy—Personally Loving Relationships,* by John H. McGoey, SFM
- *Life-Giving Love,* by Kimberly Hahn
- *Good News about Sex and Marriage: Answers to Your Honest Questions About Catholic Teaching,* by Christopher West
- *Sex and Sacredness,* by Christopher Derrick
- *New Perspectives on Contraception,* by Dr. Donald DeMarco
- Humanae Vitae *A Generation Later,* by Dr. Janet Smith
- *Why Humanae Vitae Was Right,* ed. by Dr. Janet Smith
- *Three to Get Married,* by Fulton J. Sheen
- *Catholic Sexual Ethics: A Summary, Explanation and Defense,* by Father Ronald Lawler, O.F.M. Cap, Joseph Boyle, Jr., and William E. May
- *Sex and the Marriage Covenant,* by John Kippley
- *Love & Family: Raising a Traditional Family in a Secular World,* by Mercedes Arzu Wilson
- *The Thrill of the Chaste,* by Dawn Eden

Educational Organizations

- *One More Soul*, an organization with resources galore that support families, educates about the harms of contraception, and promotes the culture of life.
  616 Five Oaks Ave.
  Dayton, OH 45406
  (800) 307-SOUL
  omsoul@omsoul.com
  In Canada: www.omsoul.ca
- *Blessed Arrows,* for financial support for couples seeking sterilization reversal. Contact www.blessedarrows.org for more information and networking avenues.
- *The Gift Foundation*
  P.O. Box 95
  Carpentersville, IL 60110
  (800) 421-GIFT
  www.giftfoundation.org
  info@giftfoundation.org
- *Life Site News*
  www.lifesitenews.ca, a daily news source on international current affairs from an orthodox Catholic perspective.
- *Human Life International,* online at http://www.hli.org, the world's largest international pro-life organization.

APPENDIX

Sexual Addiction

- *The Courage to Be Chaste,* by Benedict Groeschel, CFR
- *Impossible Joy,* by Ron J.
- *Out of the Shadows,* by Patrick Carnes, PhD
- *Feathers of the Skylark: Sin, Compulsion and Our Need for a Messiah,* by Jeffrey Satinover, MD
- *False Intimacy,* by Harry Schaumberg
- *The Porn Myth: Exposing the Reality Behind the Fantasy of Pornography,* by Matt Fradd

Marriage Counseling and Support

- *Retrouvaille*
  A very successful program for troubled marriages, even those despairing of divorce.
  http://www.retrouvaille.org
- *Marriage Encounter*
  (800) 75-LOVE
  www.wwme.org
- *Building an Outstanding Family: A Seven-Step Christian Plan,*
  by Ross Porter, PhD.
  www.stillpointfamilyresources.org
  (818) 704-9117
- *Marriage 911: God Saved Our Marriage (and Can Save Yours, Too),* by Greg and Julie Alexander
- *Loving to Fight or Fighting to Love: Winning the Spiritual Battle for Your Marriage,* by Gordon Dalbey and Mary Andrews-Dalbey

New Reproductive Technologies

- *Catholic Bioethics and the Gift of Human Life*, by William E. May
- *The Gift of Life*, by Fr. David Q. Liptak
- *On the Meaning of Sex*, by J. Budziszewski
- The United States Conference of Catholic Bishops, relevant documents all in one place: http://www.usccb.org/issues-and-action/human-life-and-dignity/reproductive-technology/index.cfm
- *Preaching Points* PDF on In Vitro Fertilization from The National Catholic Bioethics Center: https://www.ncbcenter.org/files/2614/3094/3360/IVFPreachingPoints.pdf